AF737341

Medical Outcasts

Medical Outcasts

Gendered and Institutionalized Xenophobia in Undocumented Forced Migrants' Emergency Health Care

Roxane Richter, Ph.D., E.M.T.

LEXINGTON BOOKS
Lanham • Boulder • New York • London

Published by Lexington Books
An imprint of The Rowman & Littlefield Publishing Group, Inc.
4501 Forbes Boulevard, Suite 200, Lanham, Maryland 20706
www.rowman.com

Unit A, Whitacre Mews, 26-34 Stannary Street, London SE11 4AB

British Library Cataloguing in Publication Information Available

Library of Congress Cataloging-in-Publication Data

Names: Richter, Roxane, author.
Title: Medical outcasts : gendered and institutionalized xenophobia in undocumented forced migrants' emergency health care / Roxane Richter.
Description: Lanham : Lexington Books, [2015] | Includes bibliographical references and index.
Identifiers: LCCN 2015039078 | ISBN 9781498525442 (cloth : alk. paper) | ISBN 9781498525459 (electronic)
Subjects: LCSH: Emergency medical services—Texas—Houston. | Emergency medical services—South Africa—Johannesburg. | Minority women—Medical care—United States—Houston. | Minority women—Medical care—South Africa—Johannesburg. | Discrimination in medical care. | Medical policy.
Classification: LCC RA645.6.T4 R53 2015 | DDC 362.18—dc23 LC record available at http://lccn.loc.gov/2015039078

∞™ The paper used in this publication meets the minimum requirements of American National Standard for Information Sciences—Permanence of Paper for Printed Library Materials, ANSI/NISO Z39.48-1992.

Printed in the United States of America

Dedication

This research is dedicated to Evans Tendayi Kuntonda (July 15, 1980–4 March, 2011), a passionate, humble and astute Zimbabwean activist who was a beautiful soul that worked for refugee's healthcare rights. I met Evans on my first trip to inner city of Johannesburg in 2008, where he became my inspiration to work with Zimbabwean refugees. Evans served as a Médecins Sans Frontières (MSF) community Health Promoter, building trust in order to gain access to some of the most difficult-to-reach slums. When his people suffered, he suffered. I know he provided 'fatherly' support, encouragement and role modeling for young Zimbabwean teenagers and kids who were without family, friends, and/or earthly possessions. His too-short life, for me, became the embodiment of the Zim refugee: perseverant, good-natured, forever optimistic about his homeland—but carrying a palpable sadness within; the burden of secondhand daydreams enfolded in the spoils of worn-out hope. *Vafamba zvakanaka shamwari mwari ngaakuropafadze nebasa rawakaita kuti Zimbabwe ibudirire*, dear Evans.

Contents

List of Figures ix

List of Tables xi

Acknowledgments xiii

Preface xv

1 Denial of Care 1
Feminist Perspectives and Praxis 4
Context of the Current Crises 7
Definitions and Terminology 16

2 Women in Disasters 21
Disaster Types and their Consequences for Women 27
Are Women Human? 38
More than a Uterus: Maternal Care Ethics 43

3 Asylum and Immigration 47
The Push and Pull of Migration 49
Policies of South Africa 53
Policies of the U.S.A. 58
Policy Enforcement and Litigation 63

4 Voices of the Women 69
In Their Own Words 73
Theoretical Rights vs. Practical Effects 85

5 Host Country Health Care 91
A Tale of Two Host Nations' Healthcare Systems 92
Public Health Ethics 97
Code Blue: Sustainability of Current Healthcare Systems 104

6 Women's Health 113
Pathology and Physiology of Women's Health and Disease 113
Female Migrants and Emergency Care 118
Mental Health and Gender-Based Violence 127

7 A Chance for Change 135
Gender Transformations 136
Innovative Ideas 138
Politics and Policy Creation 145
The 20-Point "Gender-Aware Disaster Care" Checklist 148

8 A Structural Violation of Human Rights 153
Cultures of Cultivation or Eradication? 154
Facing Forward 162

Appendix A: Gender, Justice, and Health Questionnaire 165

Appendix B: Zvemamiriro edu, Zvemitemo NeZveutano Mibvunzo neMhinduro 169

Appendix C: Cuestionario de género, justicia y salud 173

Appendix D: The Patients' Rights Charter – South Africa 177

Appendix E: U.S. Department of Health and Human Services "Fact Sheet"–For Patient Bill of Rights, 1999 181

Appendix F: EMTALA: Emergency Medical Treatment and Active Labor Act, 1986 189

Bibliography 197

Index 211

About the Author 213

List of Figures

Figure P.1	"Clinic Without Walls"	xvi
Figure P.2	"Queen Mother of Compassion"	xvii
Figure 3.1	Immigration Profile: South Africa	50
Figure 3.2	Immigration Profile: United States	51
Figure 4.1	Surveyed Undocumented Zimbabwean and Mexican Women—Months in Host Country	73
Figure 5.1	Major U.S. Government-Sponsored Programs and their Availability to Undocumented Immigrants	96
Figure 5.2	Adult HIV/AIDS Infection Rate Comparison in Mexico, South Africa, U.S.A., and Zimbabwe 2008	99
Figure 6.1	Conceptualization of Constrained Choice	115
Figure 6.2	Life Expectancy Comparisons 1960–2008: U.S.A., Mexico, South Africa, and Zimbabwe	116
Figure 6.3	Utilized Healthcare Services by Interviewed Zimbabwean and Mexican Women in Host Country	121
Figure 7.1	Gender-Aware Triage and Care	148
Figure 7.2	How Gender-Aware Interventions Can Reduce Impact, Acuity and Costs	151

List of Tables

Table 2.1 Galtung Violence Typology 23
Table 2.2 Gender Instruments Timeline, RSA and U.S.A. 40

Acknowledgments

Special thanks go to my fantastic son. Rainier, and doting husband, Tom, as the two people in my life who keep my footing solid, even during my unabashedly idealistic "Save the World" endeavors. I am the C.E.O. (Chief Eternal Optimist) of this biosocial feminist research and I hope it sheds some light on the current inequities in health care – the worst possible form of injustice, in my opinion. This research would not have been possible without the sage guidance and advice of Dr. Sheila Meintjes and Dr. Elias Bongmba, my stalwart backbones of brilliant and encouraging academic support. 1 am also grateful to the Bishop Dr. Paul Verryn, my friends at Central Methodist Church and Albert Street School in Johannesburg, Dr. Jose Peraza, Dr. Tom Pruett, William Kandowe, FundaciOn Rotaria de Guerrero Brigada Medica Oftalmologica, Evans Kuntonda, and all of my colleagues and co-laborers at World Missions Possible. I devote this dissertation to all of the women who continue to suffer and wait for justice and equity in health care, in politics, in economic development, in disaster aid – and even in their own homes.

Women fly when men aren't watching.

Preface

This research grew out of my firsthand experience in healthcare aid and human rights activism during the previous 15 years. In my travels to 67 countries and aid work in 16 developing nations, I have witnessed widespread inequities, injustices, and inhumanities in undocumented women's emergency healthcare access. On the frontline, my interventions as an emergency medical aid-worker gave me insight into xenophobic and gender-inequitable conditions throughout a wide range of cultures, customs, governments, and both natural and man-made disasters. This led me to the idea of developing my understanding more fully through undertaking seven years of research. I was predominantly interested in the intersections of political policy, gender studies, and emergency medical access among poor undocumented women; therefore I conceived of this biosocial social justice research project. Through this research, I hope to give voice to the unique experience of undocumented female refugees and forced migrants in seeking emergency healthcare access in host countries. Thus this research is the culmination of 24 one-on-one interviews with undocumented Mexican women in the U.S.A. and Zimbabwean women in South Africa seeking lifesaving emergency healthcare access. This theoretical and practitioner-based fieldwork shows the direct and deplorable effects of xenophobic policies coupled with a demonstrable failure to enforce healthcare access rights.

As a social justice activist among poor and oppressed women in the U.S.A. and in Africa, I am honored to be a crowned Queen Mother, "*Ama Oyemiyiefo NkƆsohemaa*" (Fante/Akan language for "Queen Mother of Compassion, Saturday-born") in Ekotsi-Bogyano, Ghana (Ekumfi Ekrawfo area, Central Region). My role as "Nana," or Queen Mother, is primarily to intercede with the chief, Nana Kwefi Arkoh, on behalf of the women and the poor of the area and seek to improve and develop women's social and fiscal

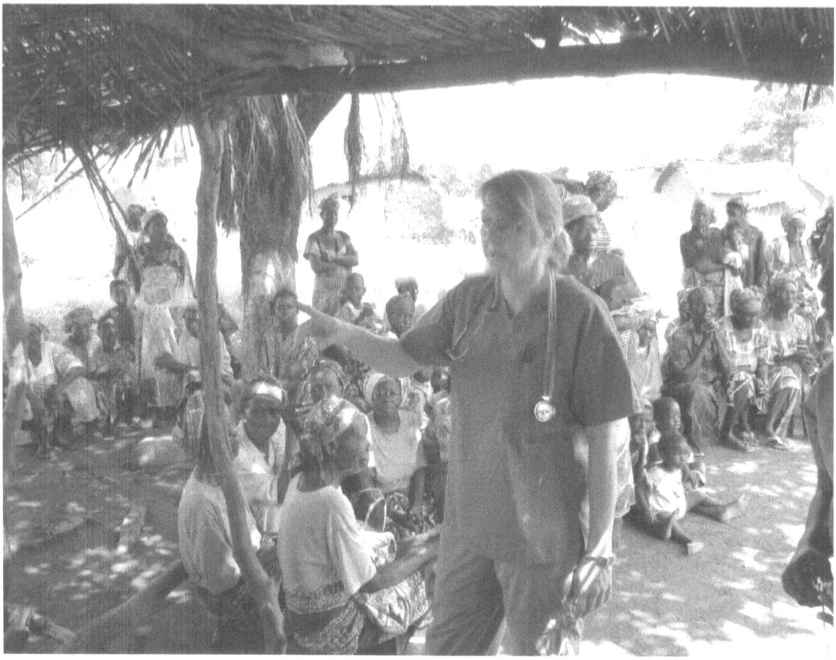

Figure P.1 Organizing Free Patient Care in African Village at an Outdoor "Clinic Without Walls."

status, as well as their access to education and health care. In this role I have witnessed firsthand how the innate bonds of sisterhood and motherhood can erase manmade boundaries or hegemonies.

Paradoxically, it was my life in Houston and my travels to Johannesburg on medical outreaches that allowed me to draw analogous parallels between the immigration influx and healthcare crises between the two burgeoning urban 'migrant mega-centers' of Houston and Johannesburg. This fateful epiphany was to serve as the catalyst for seven years of research that would inextricably tie the 'Third World' to my world. It was within these two cities that I witnessed the human worth and rights of forced migrants reduced to *political hot potatoes*—uninvited and unwanted liabilities to be hastily juggled from one government agency, hospital, or NGO's hand to another—with no one agreeably disposed to take any comprehensive responsibility or desiring any lasting ownership of the forced migrant quandary.

It was iniquitous and discriminatory policies that allowed Fungayi, a young undocumented Zimbabwean, to lose her first baby after six hours complaining of fever, vomiting, and back pain at a local Johannesburg hospital. The head nurse had shouted at her: "You are a Zimbabwean. You must go back! We are sick and tired of Zimbabweans here . . . We've been attending

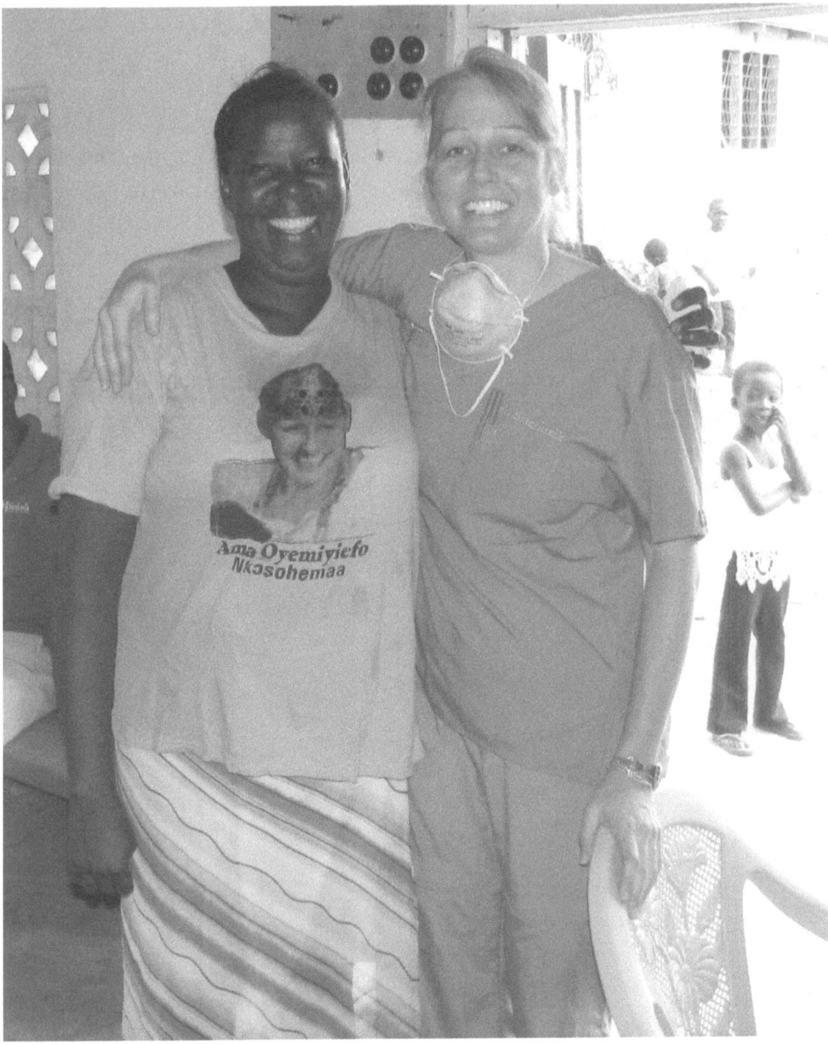

Figure P.2 Pictured (R) Providing Free Medical Eye Care at Ekotsi-Bogyano Village, where I am "Nana." "Queen Mother of Compassion"—Female Resident Wearing My Coronation Ceremony T-Shirt to Honor Me.

Zimbabweans all day!" And it was these iniquitous and discriminatory policies that led Elena, an undocumented Mexican Latina, to wait over eight hours at an emergency room, only to miscarry as she lingered among the dozens of other indigent patients in one of Houston's overcrowded public hospital emergency rooms. It is Fungayi, Elena, and many more who speak for undocumented women that report being denied emergency care, charged illegal fees, and mocked by callous healthcare staffers. This research seeks to give a voice to these women.

Working in state-sponsored organizations and NGOs as providers and activists, we fear that the continued existence of our services is contingent upon openly challenging any institutionalized xenophobic, discriminatory and/or gendered policies of the state. If left unchallenged, inequities within the ideologies of emergency preparedness planners, politicians, and healthcare institutions will continue to result in prejudice, gender-based structural violence, and inadequate and/or inequitable access to lifesaving healthcare. As activists, medical aid workers, and social scientists, we can draw not only an intangible line—but rather a palpable correlation—between a state's systematic and systemic denial of emergency health care to a structural violation of human rights.

In the end, if we are to effectively engage in the struggle for social justice and human rights, we must proactively meet the emergency healthcare needs of undocumented women by closing political loopholes, eradicating prejudicial healthcare policies, and enforcing regulations that will change today's theoretical rights into tomorrow's tangible practices.

Chapter 1

Denial of Care

"You have no papers . . . We don't assist you foreigners!" shouted the South African hospital admissions clerk at Constance, a 28-year-old Zimbabwean undocumented migrant who was two months pregnant and experiencing complications. Constance, and other undocumented refugees and forced migrants like her, are particularly vulnerable to suffer the illegal denial of care, gender discrimination, unlawful fees, xenophobic institutionalized policies, and other barriers to emergency healthcare in a host nation. Conversely, in the "American version" of care denial, a 43-year-old undocumented and uninsured Mexican woman named Zoila was told to bring—over the phone—the astronomical fee of $25,000 prior to receiving any medical attention at a private Houston-area hospital.

This transdisciplinary study—based upon qualitative biosocial, global emergency healthcare, feminist, and political science methodological pluralism—will serve to examine disparities between American and South African gendered policies and politics in emergency medical care and disaster services for undocumented (or unrecognized) refugees and forced migrants, specifically addressing women's emergency care and treatment among Mexican women in Houston, Texas, U.S.A., and Zimbabwean women in Johannesburg, South Africa. The epistemological rationale for the initial correlation of these two host countries and populations will be explained in greater detail later on in the study. However, some of the motivations are drawn from the investigation of these two refugee crises include five primary similarities. First, both the influxes of large Mexican and Zimbabwean populations into the U.S.A. and South Africa stem not from natural but rather from manmade disasters, rooted in inadequate access to food, healthcare, education, and social services, exposure to violence, and, most significantly, from national political policy challenges. Currently, Mexico's poor economy has forced Mexicans to flee severe economic hardships, drug violence, and gang murders of over 50,000 people from 2006 to 2012. Zimbabwe's economic and political meltdown resulted in a world record in hyperinflation of 231,000,000%, violence and torture, an unprecedented 95% unemployment rate in 2009, and a lack of basic commodities, but the economy has since enjoyed small rallies of 4% (2012) to 9% growth per year (2010–2011) (CIA 2013). Second, while both Mexican and Zimbabwean refugee populations can be characterized as "forced migrations," with crises that have caused displacement, extreme social and familial disruption, violence (domestic, physical and sexual), and psychosocial trauma (as defined by the WHO as a slow-onset refugee disaster), neither of these two aforementioned populations have been granted "official" refugee status by the United Nations or other internationally recognized partner. Third, both host nations possess (components of) developed emergency healthcare systems and technologically sophisticated equipment/services—whereas the majority of the poor forced migrant populations endure (components of) substandard public healthcare (in the form of immunization/wellness programs, chronic healthcare services, and so on). Fourth, both the female Mexican (Latina) and Zimbabwean populations remain at high risk for social stigmatization, subjacent social power, and subordinate value/efficacy within their own (minority) migrant culture as well as their host country's (majority) culture. Lastly, both forced migration/refugee crises are currently ongoing, and can be considered slow-onset, prolonged, manmade (not natural; human-manufactured, a result of human intent or negligence) disasters.

This transdisciplinary feminist fieldwork, explicitly partisan to social change and social justice services, uncovers the shared encounters of economic crises, large-scale "mixed" migrations, population influxes, unrecognized statuses, and emergency healthcare experiences among female Mexican undocumented Latinas in the U.S.A. and unrecognized female Zimbabwean forced migrants in South Africa. Mixed migrations like these can be defined as complex population movements that comprise refugees, asylum-seekers, economic migrants and other migrants and/or people who travel in irregular patterns (along similar routes, using similar means of travel) for dissimilar motivations (UNHCR 2015). It is through these two mutually shared and transcribed experiences that the social forces of racism, xenophobia, gender inequity, poverty, and political oppression—each a "social trigger" that prompts and propels poor healthcare access—that lead to the (direct or indirect) inequitable governance of public and personal wellness or illness.

As Paul Farmer, M.D., a prominent clinician who is noted for his research linking disease and health inequalities (molecular-basis enquiries of biological scientific realities) to poverty (psychosocial existence) noted, these "social determinants of disease" are hard to disregard when healthcare practitioners, politicians, and social scientists review the biosocial realities of the effects of power, wealth, and privilege on health. As Farmer notes:

> The disparities of risk and outcome described here are embedded in complex biosocial realities. To understand these realities, nothing less than a biosocial analysis will do—an analysis that draws freely on clinical medicine and on social theory, linking molecular epidemiology to history, ethnography, and political economy. . . . The inequalities of outcome I describe are by and large biological reflections of social fault lines. (Farmer 1999, 5)

Farmer also noted that: "One reason for this gap is that the holy grail of modern medicine remains the search for the molecular basis of disease" (Farmer et al. 2006, 44), and that this "exclusive focus on molecular-level" science "has contributed to the increasing 'desocialization' of scientific inquiry," as well as a propensity to ask "only biological questions about what are in fact *biosocial* phenomena" (Farmer et al. 2006, 44).

As for socially constructed gender-based biosocial realities, research demonstrates that women have gender-distinctive physical, psychological, social and economic needs, vulnerabilities, and opportunities in refugee and forced migration disasters. These gender-distinctive roles, behaviors, and differences manifest themselves in refugee impact, response, relief, and recovery. However, these gender-based differences have yet to be fully researched, studied, and exploited. The 2002 World Health Organization's *Gender and Health in Disasters* report revealed that there is a lack of research on sex and gender differences in vulnerabilities and impacts of disasters like refugee mass migrations. But these preliminary studies suggest that there is a pattern of gender differentiation at all levels of both natural and manmade disasters. This is broken down into exposure to risk, risk perception, preparedness, response, physical impact, psychological impact, recovery, and reconstruction (WHO 2002).

While this transdisciplinary biosocial research does not attempt to study emergency healthcare access in host countries among recognized refugees, documented migrants, or (foreign-born) naturalized citizens, it does seek to study female migrants that are considered undocumented, forced, or illegal immigrants without legal migration status in either the South Africa (Zimbabwean-born refugees or forced migrants) or the U.S.A. (Mexican-born refugees or forced migrants) who have sought out emergency healthcare. This research will attempt not only to identify issues, but to call attention to proactive interventions like female-specific emergency healthcare supplies and triage services, "gender-aware" needs assessments, crisis support intervention, as well as public healthcare and wellness advocacy. This research makes the supposition that not gender—*but gender inequity*—is the mechanism that places girls and women at heightened risks before, during, and after manmade and natural disasters. It is this acute segregation (or "otherness") in social, political, and economic power; cultural roles; and social frameworks that trigger and ignite the firestorms of structural violence, biosocial, and constructed vulnerabilities.

FEMINIST PERSPECTIVES AND PRAXIS

Within this feminist epistemological research, it is my hope that several significant lessons can be learned in the area of gender justice, power relations, humanitarianism, and female-specific undocumented migrant emergency healthcare access. A feminist research epistemology was employed in this research since feminism's most engaging and persuasive epistemological insight is considered by many noted feminist scholars (Doucet and Mauthner 2006, Lennon and Whitford 1994) as the correlation between constructs of knowledge and power. That being said, Sandra Harding has noted that the logic of "standpoint epistemologists" (and feminists who employ this kind of theory of knowledge) "start thought with marginalized lives" and then "takes everyday life as problematic" (1993, 51). Thus, this feminist research employs not only correlations between power differentials and healthcare access/wellness issues, but also other feminist methodology, method, or epistemology characteristics as noted by Doucet and Mauthner (2006), including concerns with social change and social justice; inequitable power relations/power hierarchy between the researcher and his or her researched subjects; and finally, that feminist research is not only *about* women, but *for* women (and, whenever possible, *with* women). As for the challenges associated with multicultural feminist research, Behar adeptly notes the researcher must negotiate the multilingual and transdisciplinary spheres of academia, feminist solidarity, and in this specific case, the additional realms of political science and emergency medical policies and practice. Thus some of today's modern-day feminist scholars don the role of "witness" as a key form of tackling and transforming our present-day realities (Behar 1996) and shine a penetrating light on those socially unjust and discriminatory "dark places" (Watson 2009, 1). Denzin concurs with Behar that feminist field research has a distinct commitment to a "social justice agenda"—adding a "political component" so that inequities and injustices in specified social movements (like xenophobia and gender justice) and geographic areas (like South Africa and the United States) are explicitly defined through interpretive ethnographies in time(s) and place(s) (2014, p. x). Additionally, it should be noted that feminist research is based on a few "collectively accepted" assumptions, according to Sotirios Sarantokos, including that the world is "socially constructed," embraces a distinct opposition to empirical positivistic methodology, and rejects "value-free nature of research," yet utilizes qualitative and/

or quantitative methodologies, albeit adjusting quantitative methodologies in order to fulfill requisites within the feminist archetype (2012, 54). Yet despite its feminist contributions, there are particular sensitivities and convictions concerning poststructuralism and neopositivistic empiricism in feminist fieldwork, Kim England notes:

> Feminism and the so-called postmodern turn in the social sciences represent a serious challenge to the methodological hegemony of neopositivist empiricism. One of the main attractions of "traditional" neopositivist methods is that they provide a firmly anchored epistemological security from which to venture out and conduct research. Neopositivist empiricism specifies a strict dichotomy between object and subject as a prerequisite for objectivity. Such an epistemology is supported by methods that position the researcher as an omnipotent expert in control of both passive research subjects and the research process. . . . The neopositivist's professional armor includes a carefully constructed public self as a mysterious, impartial outsider, an observer free of personality and bias. (England 1994, 242)

Correspondingly, this piece of research employs Sarantokos' theories on feminist research as a purposive quest that can be transdisciplinary, places emphasis on women's experiences (which are considered key indicators of oppressive realities), includes the researcher as a person, is "politically value-laden and critical" (not methodological but dialectical), plus is "contextual, inclusive, involved, socially relevant . . . not necessarily replicable, open to the environment, and inclusive of emotions and events as experienced" (2012, 55–56). Similarly, Richa Nagar and Susan Geiger note the exceptional and singular qualities proffered by transdisciplinary feminist research:

> Transdisciplinary feminist scholarship can support and facilitate collective and collaborative international research, and take the lead in redefining the relationship between scholarship and community-based "service" and how academic merit gets valued. It can be critical in moving us beyond the impasse by creating institutional spaces promoting a far broader view of what counts as significant scholarship, and by encouraging graduate students and faculty to take intellectual and political risks—including the highly charged and thoroughly scrutinized practice known as feminist fieldwork. (Nagar and Geiger 2007, 16)

Succinctly put, feminist fieldwork and research like this transdisciplinary examination anticipates the construction of significant contributions to mainstream, alternative, academic, and fieldwork considerations about power relations, representation, and feminist enquiry—and is driven by, and aimed toward, a desire to challenge multiple hierarchies or inequalities within social life (Doucet and Mauthner 2006). Furthermore, the transformation of social life and the pursuit of social justice are key central canons of feminist research enquiry (Hesse-Biber and Yaiser 2004). Feminist enquiry therefore maintains that research is inherently and instinctively a political endeavor—positioned as per *the personal is political*—seeking to "interrogate power relations in the production of knowledge" (Somekh and Lewin 2011). This "personal is political" consciousness-raising women's liberation catchphrase from the 1960s and 1970s serves to underscore how issues in women's personal lives (e.g. access to healthcare, sexual assault) is essentially a political matter (vis-à-vis oppressive and systemic group struggle and institutionalized structural inequities). Ideally, the catalysts behind this woman's-lib phrase is to inspire and empower women to become more politically active and to compel politics and politicians to enact legislation that advanced gender justice for a collective/unified pro-woman action that would bring about a collective/unified pro-woman solution (Hanisch 1969).

Considering the international feminist geopolitics engaged in this particular research, Behar noted that no one has a conclusive reconciliation of feminist politics (i.e. social transformation and international sisterhood) with that of a research project pertaining to (privileged) academic women recording and publishing (underprivileged) women from "somewhere else in the name of a feminism to be borne across the border" (1993, 297). It was noted American feminism and post-colonial theorist Sandra Harding who is credited with the concept of sanctioning and "privileging" typically (and traditionally) silenced and/or subjugated voices of women (consortiums of women who are customarily repressed) in the production of knowledge (1987). So the voices of these (politically and socially muted) undocumented Mexican and Zimbabwean women—as a subjugated and traditionally "silenced" group proffer a unique, valuable, and distinctive array of experiences that have been conventionally overlooked in the production of academic knowledge (Somekh and Lewin 2011). Like so many before me, the feminist fieldworker struggles with negotiating international borders, especially those between first- and third-world groups (Nagar and Geiger 2007). Thus, Nagar and Geiger point out the significance of identifying what geopolitical borders (and whose interests?) are traversed, and how these observations may be tinged with ideologies of imperialism, Western knowledge (first-world values), and neo-colonialism (2007). Therefore, this transdisciplinary research positions itself within the realm of feminist participatory fieldwork to observe and examine the effects of constructed "social determinants" or "social origins" of suffering, disease, wellness, and emergency healthcare access—such as gender inequity, structural violence, barriers to access, human rights, political flux, and more—within these two specified groups of women.

Another enquiry this study strives to address is the impact of gender, civil, humanitarianism, and social justice politics and healthcare policies on undocumented Zimbabwean women's emergency care in South Africa (with its Constitution-based rights to emergency healthcare under a dual public and private healthcare system)—when considered alongside undocumented Mexican women's emergency care in the U.S.A. (with its "Good Samaritan" policies and newly mandated "Obamacare")? Accordingly, this study will provide a broad-spectrum outline of American and South African human rights, immigration, disaster, and gender-based policies that comprise legal mandates and emergency medical aid (e.g. triage indices and gender-based biology) directives that set the parameters for emergency healthcare services afforded to these two specified groups in their host countries. To further explore this topic, the role of government in shaping these systemic and institutionalized ideologies, constructs and tenets will be examined, as well as selected public paradigms that effect national healthcare expenditures, subsidized programs, public health risks, and humanitarian intervention (e.g. aid, power relations/sovereignty, and the "politics of compassion"). As social scientist Didier Fassin observes: "Compassion represents the most complete manifestation of this paradoxical combination of heart and reason," in that the "sympathy felt for the misfortune of one's neighbor generates the moral indignation that can prompt action to end it" (2012, 1).

Ultimately the contribution and intention of this study is not to provide definitive recommendations of specific forced migration policies that have a civic and/or partisan duty to be executed, but rather to serve as a poignant and personal illustration of how particular social tenets, inequitable power relations, and political economy subjugation can and do directly impact socioeconomically disadvantaged women's health, livelihood, gender justice, and human rights.

CONTEXT OF THE CURRENT CRISES

The political and economic conditions in Zimbabwe and Mexico that have led to such mass migrations have both taken place over prolonged periods of time: In Zimbabwe, the regime of Robert Mugabe began to wreak economic, social, and political havoc back in 1980; in Mexico, residents have continued to struggle for decades against crime, economic hardships, and the violent rule of drug cartels. In brief, Zimbabwe's political and economic history since independence: Mugabe came to power as Prime Minister in 1980 after the Lancaster House agreement, and he retained the Westminster model until 1989, making himself executive President or effective one-party rule. In June 2007, Mugabe instituted price controls on all basic commodities causing panic-buying and Zimbabweans were mired in unrelenting violence, soaring inflation, hunger, destitution, lawlessness, and all the while the country's health system had all but disintegrated, schools were in dire straits, and most public services had collapsed (Meredith 2007). Much of the fate of the country's current state of social and, economic, and political repression must be shouldered by the regime of Robert Mugabe, who was elected president of Zimbabwe in 1980, and led the Zimbabwe African National Union—Patriotic Front (ZANU-PF) regime. According to Meredith: "Year after year, Mugabe sustained his rule through violence and repression—crushing political opponents, violating the courts, trampling on property rights, suppressing the independent press, and rigging elections" (2007, 18). By the year 2000, Zimbabweans were worse off than they had been at independence in 1980: average wages were lower, unemployment had tripled, public services were crumbling, and life expectancy was falling. For Meredith, "It was as if Mugabe and his inner circle had come to regard Zimbabwe as the spoils of war, for their own use" (Meredith 2007, 17). These issues forced millions of Zimbabweans to flee the political violence and economic crises in Zimbabwe and search for jobs, health, social, and public services in neighboring countries, such as South Africa. Research by Human Rights Watch (2008) shows that since 2005 over 1.5 million Zimbabweans (out of a 13 million population in 2013) have fled across the 225-kilometer border shared with South Africa in order to escape repression, political persecution, forced evictions, and economic destitution, and to seek food, shelter, employment, and healthcare. In 2008, annual inflation in Zimbabwe hit an estimated 96 sextillion percent—96,000,000,000,000,000,000,000%, according to a February 2013 CNN report. Current 2013 studies show the World Bank ranks this country as number 172 (out of 185) for "ease of doing business," and number 163 (out of 174) in the world's corruption rankings by global watchdog group, Transparency International (CNN). The endemic and systemic epidemic that is exterminating the country's wealth it seems is corruption in the political, private, and civil sectors. After the 2008 elections, Mugabe and ZANU-PF controlled over 14 critical ministries (including defense, home and foreign affairs, justice, media, mines, and land). The role of Prime Minister was re-established to accommodate the MDC, yet gave Morgan Tsvangirai, the leader of the MDC little real power. Meanwhile, the ZANU-PF party and Mugabe's subordinates tolerated and sanctioned millions and billions in national revenue to disappear from the country's coffers. Evidence for this is widespread, but a case in point is that in November 2011, a Canadian watchdog group alleged that more than 2 billion dollars' worth of diamonds had "gone missing" since 2008. In February 2013, the country's finance minister, Tendai Biti, disclosed that the entire country had only 217 U.S. dollars in its public account. Biti also disclosed that Zimbabwe's mining sector produced $2.5 billion in exports in 2011 alone—but only 6%, some $150 million, actually found its way into the country's public treasury. With 94% of Zimbabwe's mining revenue in 2011 "unaccounted for" and the finance minister shrugging his shoulders as to the whereabouts of the country's wealth, there is little confidence among multinational corporations interested in investing in Zimbabwe's future. Despite such dire reports on corruption, hyperinflation and dubious incidents, since April 12, 2009, Zimbabwe adopted the U.S. dollar as legal tender, which halted the hyperinflation and somewhat stabilized the economy. According to the International Monetary Fund, the country's Gross Domestic Product (GDP) grew more than 6% in 2009, almost 10% in 2010 and 2011, and is on course for a projected annual 5% growth through year 2014 (CNN 2013). In a country where the national per capita income is about $1 a day—yet the leader lavished $1 million on his 88th birthday party—it is clear that obliterating rampant political, civil, judicial, and private corruption, poor governance, and organized crime will be difficult to achieve. Yet the key to change lies in creating a culture of democratic accountability and commitment of the political class to the well-being of the population. The country has considerable social capital, and its economic infrastructure was once sound. Thus there is a basis upon which unlocking the potential and wealth of this struggling country can proceed. Zimbabwe must seek to form and enforce a nation-wide strategy to combat corruption in order to foster effective, transparent, participatory, and responsive governance. Perhaps the state of corruption in Zimbabwe is best articulated by a native Zimbabwean himself. In the *New Zimbabwe*, Tonderai Munakiri had this to say about the aspects of corruption in his home country:

> Power has corrupted our governors and the absolute power they wield has made them more gluttonous. The young generations aspiring for political office in our midst are no longer driven by a sense of servitude but by the gains of the office that they would occupy. . . . The visions that were espoused at independence have all become pipedreams and nightmares; we have lost the Zimbabwean dream. (Munakiri 2009, 1)

In his February 3, 2013, CNN Global Public Square reporter Fareed Zakaria stated that Zimbabwe "has gone from Africa's breadbasket to its basket case." And after 10 years of economic destruction, Zimbabwe was recently rated as the "second-worst" failed state in the world by *Foreign Policy*, just behind Somalia (Horne 2009).

Similar to the desire of some Zimbabwean citizens to regain their country's stable economy and loosen its dictator's political stranglehold, Mexico's population are equally determined to fight crime and elude its vice-like grip of violence. Mexico has been a developing country struggling against drug trafficking, organized crime, corruption, and economic hardships for several decades. Some of the country's ongoing economic hardships can be traced back to specific events such as the 1982 devaluation of the national currency (peso) by 78%, and then the 1994–1995 "Mexican Peso Crisis," an event that triggered the country's worst depression in 60 years. Current 2013 reports show the World Bank ranks Mexico 48th (out of 185) for "ease of doing business," and 105th (out of 176) in the world's corruption rankings in 2012 by the German global watchdog group, Transparency International. The apparent inability of the national police and military force to control the flow of guns and violence continues to suppress anti-crime efforts, to rattle the nerves of Americans situated along Mexican-American border, and to bring into question if the $1.4 billion in U.S. anticrime aid is beneficial in ending, or even stemming, the country's relentless bloodshed. Despite these and other efforts, organized crime in Mexico's "Drug War" continues to skyrocket. Since Mexico's President Felipe Calderón began his push against gun-running and drug cartels between 2006 and 2012, more than 60,000 people have died in a string of violent shootouts, bombings, and murders. For example in May 2012, some 49 bodies—without heads, hands or feet—were discovered in trash bags on a highway in northern Mexico, reported *The Atlantic*, a Washington, D.C.-based newspaper (Taylor 2012).

The drug war in Mexico not only claims the lives of organized crime members—but also the lives of police and journalists. In July 2008, drug-related crimes had caused the death of over 170 police officers (Debusmann 2008). Media coverage of drug crime and trafficking led to the death of 81 and the disappearance of 14 reporters since 2000, with one gang sending the decapitated head of a murdered journalist to his newsroom as a warning according to Paris-based Reporters without Borders (2008). These episodes of torture, oppression, murder, and kidnapping among Mexican reporters have made the country the most dangerous country in the Western hemisphere. In the world, Mexico is ranked (with Iraq) as the 2nd "most dangerous country" in the world for a journalist, outranked only by Pakistan, according to a 2010 Reporters without Borders report. The impunity rate, or percentage rate at which crimes go unsolved by a government, among Mexican journalist homicides is 98%, and is considered a key indicator of freedom of the press. The experience of journalists in Mexico could lead to self-censorship among the press corps, according to Reporters without Borders (2013). It should be noted that some of the blame for these deaths have also been leveled at Mexican police, politicians, and police force, tied to alleged corruption and negligence. In a bold move on December 10, 2008, ARTICLE 19-Mexico (an independent human rights organization that promotes the right to freedom of expression and takes its name from Article 19 of the Universal Declaration of Human Rights) and the National Center for Social Communication (CENCOS, a Mexico-based human rights organization) published a survey blaming the authorities for 49% of the physical attacks on journalists and media in

2010 with only 26% ascribed to organized crime (CENCOS 2011). The two organizations launched a campaign to protect journalists who were reporting human rights abuses and informing the public about the state of the world. The campaign slogan was: "*Te hace daño no saber*" (translated means: "What you don't know *can* hurt you") to protect journalists in Mexico:

> Every time information of public interest is withdrawn because of violence, threats or fears, it is a little piece of our humanity that is taken away. Whenever opinions, expression and information are torn, what makes us human is torn as well. . . . Journalists are under fire because of the work they do. . . . Their presence has become uncomfortable for drug cartels, police and authorities up to the federal level. . . . The core demands have to come from within. (CENCOS and ARTICLE 19-Mexico, on the 60th anniversary of the Universal Declaration of Human Rights, December 10, 2008)

These events and issues have forced many Mexicans to flee crime, violence, and economic hardships in Mexico and search for jobs, healthcare, and public services in the U.S.A., which shares a common 2,000-mile border with Mexico.

This research employed methodological pluralism to examine biosocial "social determinants" of disease, wellness, and emergency healthcare access within two stipulated groups of women (undocumented Zimbabwean women in Johannesburg, South Africa, and undocumented Mexican women in Houston, Texas, U.S.A.). It is focused on the access to emergency healthcare only among undocumented women forced migrants in their host nations. This study seeks to examine only female migrants that are considered undocumented, forced, or illegal immigrants without legal migration status in either the South Africa (Zimbabwean migrants) or the U.S.A. (Mexican Latina migrants) who have sought out emergency healthcare only, not including any long-term and/or chronic healthcare interventions. For the purposes of this research, we will define a chronic illness as a condition that usually lasts 12 months or longer and places limitations on self-care and independent living, and/or causes the need for ongoing treatment with medical products, services, and/or specialized medical equipment.

Even in countries like South Africa and the United States that provide public emergency healthcare services and access, undocumented female Zimbabwean and Mexican forced migrants can fail to benefit from these services for a variety of reasons. Language barriers, illiteracy, and poor communication between migrants and the host nation's healthcare providers are certainly observable causes (and ostensibly not within the exclusive domain of women). But how women in the forced migrant communities perceive their health and their decision-making power to affect it—remain prominent variables. Undocumented female migrants can harbor fear, superstition, trepidation, and gross misperceptions about immigration risks and their legal emergency healthcare provisions in a host country's healthcare system—and consequently resort to accessing healthcare only in extremely dire, and hence potentially life-threatening, circumstances. Logistical issues such as a lack of transportation, funds, or knowledge of local area healthcare facilities and providers can also be barriers to forced migrants' effective and timely healthcare access. So when host countries fail to empower female migrant communities with the knowledge of their legal rights to emergency healthcare, it is akin to relinquishing the undocumented refugee's or forced migrant's right to healthcare at all.

This research has attempted to not only identify relevant female emergency healthcare disaster (refugee/forced migrant) issues, but to emphasize interventions like female-specific supplies and services, "gender-aware" needs assessments, crisis support intervention, and advocacy. This work also aspires to bridge the current chasm of gender-disaggregated data, helping to uncover gender-based behavioral differences and harness and positively exploit those missed opportunities in women's undocumented forced migration disaster Emergency Medical Services (EMS) planning, mitigation, response, and recovery. The sampling and methodological pluralism chosen for this work include theoretical and literature research, fieldwork, a human research ethics examination, interviews with healthcare providers, and healthcare interviews among a group of 24 female Mexican and Zimbabwean refugees/migrants who had sought and utilized emergency healthcare services as unrecognized refugees. These interviews will hopefully provide useful insight into the women's experiences, as well as gender-based information essential for scholarly study and mainstream public media attention. The interviews involved one-on-one anonymous snowball sampling interviews with female refugees who have previously accessed or attempted to access emergency healthcare services in Houston and Johannesburg only.

The "Gender, Social Justice, and Healthcare Interview" (Appendix A—in English, Shona and Spanish languages) queries are targeted to ascertain the six following dimensions of women's experiences concerning: (1) a woman's active or passive role as a decision-maker in seeking and obtaining emergency medical care for herself; (2) assessment of realized, potential, and/or perceived physical, financial, physiological, informational, mental, and social barriers to obtaining and receiving EMS care as an unrecognized refugee or undocumented forced migrant; (3) their assessment of accessibility, availability, quality, equity (or any discrimination or discriminatory practices, such as excessive fees, racism, etc.), and credibility of EMS care and treatment; (4) their usage of the healthcare services, delineated between illnesses (diseases) and injuries (trauma-related), as well as major categories of medical practices (obstetrics, oncology, surgery, pharmaceutical, respiratory, etc.); (5) their assessment of EMS and healthcare provider response (as effective or non-effective) and treatment (respect, courtesy, xenophobia, etc.); and (6) each woman's assessment of gender-equitable and fair treatment in triage and screening processes, EMS, healthcare aid distribution, counseling, and more. The interviews themselves were conducted on a personal one-to-one basis, with only women who have personally received or attempted to receive emergency healthcare services participating in the three-page, 23-question interview, which was written in a simple (elementary/primary school) reading level of English and translated into Shona and Spanish. This research's interviews demonstrated that while theoretical healthcare rights and practical (evidence-based) healthcare rights affirm commonly shared goals—the reality lies somewhere between the two. Indubitably, theory, and evidence are neither irreconcilable nor diametrically opposed, and there are theory-guided evidence-based practices that integrate both approaches successfully, especially within the field of medical practice. But the reality of many undocumented forced migrants' experiences in claiming their accorded healthcare rights remained primarily theoretical, and not practical, in its nature. This holds true with the majority of the undocumented Zimbabwean and Mexican women I interviewed for this particular research.

To delve further into this research subject, fundamental enquiries concerning women in disasters—women's socially constructed roles, and impacts, vulnerabilities, and capabilities—will be addressed in the following (second) chapter. This will establish a formative cornerstone in an attempt to identify the construction of structural violence, gender equity, ethics of care, human capabilities, and mechanisms of social construction. Structural violence—which refers to the social consequences of society or a state's inability to fulfill an individual's needs in the context of deep structural inequities—will be defined, illustrated, and clarified. The chapter will also address variable types of disasters, their impact on women, specific causes and consequences of disaster vulnerability, as well as the current lack of gender-disaggregated data and its effect on gender equity and gendered marginalization in disasters, economic activity, political development, aid and healthcare. It seeks to address the issue of women's human rights and will compile a gender rights "timeline" that will establish analytical instruments of evaluate gender-equity-driven efforts. The chapter will conclude with a discussion of the core debates of the "ethics of care," offering a critical analysis of maternal ethics of care, and the idea of women's role as society's caregivers.

Since this research only addresses women without legal migration status in either the South Africa (Zimbabwean migrants) or the U.S.A. (Mexican migrants) who have sought out emergency healthcare, there are definitive requisites to address particularly relevant international, regional, and national laws and treatises that address rights to asylum and healthcare access to these particular groups of undocumented women. Hence, in the third chapter, several undocumented migrants' issues will be addressed, including local (state), regional, federal, and international asylum and immigration treatises pertaining to South Africa and the United States; the constructive and negative "pushes and pulls" of migration in host countries; policy enforcement and litigation; vicissitudes in gender-based asylum jurisprudence cases; and migratory populations' return to their country of origin for healthcare. Then the current and future trends in South African and American policy development vis-à-vis healthcare rights, asylum, enforcement, and litigation will be undertaken.

Voices of the Women, Chapter 4, comprises a more comprehensive framework of the purposive interviews undertaken for this research. The chapter will first investigate the methodologies used in undertaking the 24 interviews. The interviews were constructed around a "Gender, Social Justice, and Healthcare Interview" agenda (Appendix A) that sought to explore six dimensions in the experience of undocumented refugees. The six dimensions of the queries were targeted to discover decision-making roles in seeking emergency medical care; barriers to care; assessments of accessibility, availability, quality, equity, and the credibility of care; usage of the services; provider response; and gender-equitable treatment throughout the process. The second section provides a narrative analysis of the some of the firsthand accounts (i.e., the voices of the women). In this section, the narrative provides both direct and indirect quotations from the experience of the women obtained during their interviews. The third section will assess the limitations of the interviews and any significant lessons gleaned from creating and executing the various interview sessions. The final section of the chapter addresses the chasm between theoretical healthcare rights and the practical effects. While in terms of constitutional rights, undocumented refugees have (some) healthcare rights, the reality is that they were oftentimes unable to realize those rights in practice.

The ensuing fifth Host Country Healthcare chapter will review how the application of social justice shapes the tangible foundation of public healthcare in both South Africa and the United States. We will explore how it is within the realm of each country's policy makers and healthcare institution's procedures to resolve either to passively "cultivate" or actively "eradicate" the structural violence of engendered xenophobia. Our initial analysis will begin by taking an overarching national view of the core concepts, functions, primary goals, and evaluations that set up the parameters for these two host countries' healthcare systems—such as nationally mandated patient rights, constitutional provisions for healthcare access, as well as current battles being waged against pandemics and infectious/communicable diseases. Then similarities and differences between American and South African "gatekeeper" triage indexes will be studied, paralleled, and interpreted. The fiscal sustainability of both countries' current state of intense medical inflation of public and private healthcare system costs will be reviewed in section four. The final section of the chapter will report on the current state of American and South African healthcare reform, including the universal "Obamacare" (Affordable Care Act) rollout in the U.S. and the boost to South Africa's emergency care that arose from national reforms and EMS initiatives emerging from the 2010 FIFA World Cup.

Chapter 6 will analyze how women may suffer from many of the same diseases and illnesses as men—but they endure them uniquely as women within their unique physiological and psychosocial variations, constructions, and contexts. The purpose of this chapter is to explain the biological variations in women's physiological makeup, thereby delineating the link between the biological and social vulnerabilities of women in disaster and refugee situations. The "pathology and physiology of women's health and disease," gender-based biology, and pharmaceutical and toxicological variations between the sexes, will be reviewed. Studying sex-based health differences can yield greater insight into understanding biological disease mechanisms, leading, in turn, to improved treatments and outcomes (Levy and Sidel 2005). Female migration, sex differences in migration patterns, Gender-Based Violence (GBV), and rape utilized as a "weapon of war" will also be examined.

The "Chance for Change" chapter will provide an overview of selected pioneering policies that have actually accomplished positive transformation, and will then make some constructive proposals for implementation that could be transformative. Thus the seventh chapter will explore progressive changes that can take place in gender/social relations following a disaster or forced migration, and consider possible innovations that create more resourceful tools and successful protocols. To that end, I have compiled a 20-point "Gender-Aware Support and Services Checklist" of provisions, services, and aids that explicitly help to address and reduce impact, acuity and costs in post-disaster healthcare provisioning, including high gender input throughout all stages of planning, preparedness, response, recovery and reconstruction efforts; a women's "Principal Point of Contact" Resource Area; private, enclosed OB/GYN assessment and care area; daily prenatal nutritional advocacy; rape intake provisioning; "fact sheets" on potential effects of vaccines, environmental toxins and exposures on pregnancies and post-disaster onset/symptoms/treatment environmental contamination/toxic shock syndrome; and feminine hygiene kits, etc. It can be hypothesized that the stockpiling and provision of these gender-aware supplies and services could serve to decrease the risk for adverse pregnancy and infant outcomes, recurrent healthcare costs and concerns, as well as reducing requirements for multiple medical interventions.

Chapter 8 will point to some of the interviewed women's suffering as the direct and deplorable consequence of today's current gendered and xenophobic institutionalized public policies, coupled with a failure to enforce healthcare access rights. As activists, medical aid workers, and political science researchers, we can draw not only an intangible line but rather a palpable correlation between a state's systematic and systemic denial of emergency healthcare to a structural violation of human rights. Lastly, we will examine aforementioned and previously studied ideologies and policies that can directly or indirectly cultivate or eradicate xenophobia, social injustice, and gender inequity.

In conclusion, two causal points should be emphasized. First, gender-based disaster aid research and advocacy are not zero-sum games in which every word written about female suffering or indeed support for women, leads to one less word written about male suffering or means less support for men or vice versa. As a community-encompassing EMS providers, humanitarians, social scientists, and disaster aid workers, we need to seek to expose, examine, and exploit gender-based disaster issues and take appropriate actions that can potentially lead to reductions in *all* human suffering and loss. Secondly, I do not condone nor suggest that men remain unaffected by disasters, rather I hope that this research will serve as a filtered "gender lens," showing how men and women are (both) constrained by their socialization and differently, nonetheless disproportionately, impacted by disasters.

DEFINITIONS AND TERMINOLOGY

Biopolitics—a theory constructed by Michel Foucault about modern society's transition. Foucault argues that modern power differs fundamentally from sovereign power: Whereas sovereign power is categorized by a right over life and death ("killing or letting live"), modern power is characterized by "fostering life or disallowing it" (University of Memphis 2013, 1). Giorgio Agamben theorises biopolitics a little differently. He suggests that biopolitics moves natural life (*zoe*) into the "sphere of the polis" and that "natural life begins to be included in the mechanisms and calculations of State power, and politics turns into biopolitics" so life (goods *and* natural life) is a political matter (University of Memphis 2013).

Biosocial research—I refer to this research as a "biosocial" work, which extracts and entwines components of political economy, medical research, and social theory as compulsory and intrinsically intermingled elements of healthcare and disaster outcomes. This is a term coined by Paul Farmer in his book *Infections and Inequalities*, whereby he explains that "biosocial analysis draws freely on clinical medicine and on social theory, linking molecular epidemiology to history, ethnography, and political economy" (1999, 5).

Comorbidity/Comorbid disease(s)—a comorbid disease pertains to a disease or other pathological process that occurs simultaneously with another, as defined by the Miller-Keane Encyclopedia and Dictionary of Medicine, Nursing, and Allied Health (2003).

Disaster—six principal categories of disasters includes: rapid-onset disasters (such as earthquakes and storms); slow-onset disasters (such as drought and desertification); human-induced disasters (such as armed conflict); epidemics (such as HIV/AIDS); floods; and refugee emergencies (such as mass persecution, forced migration and armed conflict) according to the UN Development Program (Mocellin et al. 1994). Within the category of "refugee emergencies" is the sub-category of "forced migration" which includes three primary classifications of conflict-, disaster- and development-induced displacements (FMO 2010).

Emergency healthcare—an injury or illness that poses an immediate threat to a person's life or long-term health. There are critical care thresholds and criteria that distinguish between "emergency" (lifesaving) and other medically determined states such as "routine," "chronic," "non-emergency," and "elective" care. The patient's state, defined by pre-determined and set medical protocols, can profoundly affect a patient's receipt of care (especially that of undocumented/unrecognized or "illegal" refugees or forced migrants) under the statues of a "receiving" (or host) country's healthcare triage index and/or institution regulations for patient identification and care parameters.

EMS—refers specifically to necessary emergency pre-hospital care received by paramedical personnel in public or private ambulance service or any pre-hospital/accident/trauma scenario out-of-hospital setting.

Emergency medicine—for the purposes of this research, it is defined as a medical specialty concerned with the care and treatment of acutely ill or injured patients who need immediate medical attention.

Gender—the term "gender" refers to the socially constructed roles, behaviors, activities, and attributes that a given society considers appropriate for men and women, whereas the term "sex" refers to the biological and physiological characteristics that define men and women.

GBV—as defined in 1993 by the UN Declaration on the Elimination of Violence against Women, the first official definition of the term "GBV" is as follows: "Any act of GBV that results in, or is likely to result in, physical, sexual, or psychological harm or suffering to women, including threats of such acts, coercion or arbitrary deprivations of liberty, whether occurring in public or in private life" (HHRI 2012).

Migration—a process of social change where an individual or group for reasons of economic betterment, political upheaval, education or other purposes, leaves one geographical area (trans-national or rural-urban) for a prolonged stay in another (Bhugra and Jones 2001).

Forced migration—refers to the movements of refugees and internally displaced people (those displaced by conflicts) as well as people displaced by natural or environmental disasters, chemical or nuclear disasters, famine, or development projects, according to the International Association for the Study of Forced Migration (2010).

Postionality—the state, locus, or "position" of the researcher within his/her research, including, but not limited to, the researcher's class (status), gender, age, sexual identity, race (ethnicity), and education—all of which can serve to either impede or empower particular research fieldwork insights and methodologies.

Public health (welfare)—is defined as the science and practice of protecting and improving the health of a community, as by preventive medicine, health education, control of communicable diseases, application of sanitary measures, and monitoring of environmental hazards, according to the American Heritage Dictionary (2013).

Refugee—a person who has a well-founded fear of being persecuted on account of race, religion, nationality, membership of a particular social group, or political opinion, is outside the country of their nationality, and is unable to or owing to such fear, is unwilling to avail him/herself of the protection of that country, or a person who flees a war or other violence in their home country.

Strategic gender interests (Moser Framework)—this refers to interventions that tackle fundamental issues related to women's subordination and/or gender inequities. Strategic gender interests are long term, generally not based on material goods, and are often associated to status, power, and/or equity (structural) transformations in society, such as equal-rights legislation, reproductive choice, and increased participation in (political, economic, and social) decision-making functions. The term "strategic gender needs" was first coined by Maxine Molyneux in 1985. Molyneaux's work in strategic gender needs assisted in developing gender planning and policy development tools like the Moser Framework, a planning methodology aimed at the emancipation of women from their subordination and their achievement of equality, equity, and empowerment (World Bank 2012).

Structural violence—refers to systematic ways in which social structures harm or otherwise disadvantage or discriminate against individuals. In sharp contrast to behavioral violence, structural violence can be rather subtle, sometimes even invisible, and normally cannot be specifically identified or responsible by a person(s). The term, as defined by medical anthropologist Dr. Paul Farmer, stands as:

> Structural violence is one way of describing social arrangements that put individuals and populations in harm's way. . . . The arrangements are structural because they are embedded in the political and economic organization of our social world; they are violent because they cause injury to people . . . neither culture nor pure individual will is at fault; rather, historically given (and often economically driven) processes and forces conspire to constrain individual agency. Structural violence is visited upon all those whose social status denies them access to the fruits of scientific and social progress. (Farmer 2004, 306)

Structuralism/structures—national and international structures take many forms, and according to Landman's structuralist analysis, focus on the "holistic aspects of society, including interdependent relationships among individuals, collectives, institutions, and/or organizations" but, unlike rationalism, it contends that individuals and states do not make decisions exclusively on rational choice or selection (2006, 45). Political and economic structures include class, class coalitions, business organizations, political parties, and global institutions like the UN, World Trade Organization (WTO), and the General Agreement on Tariff and Trades (GATT), whereas social structures include sexism and racism, and class-based structures.

Undocumented, unrecognized or illegal migrant/refugee—refers to foreign-born individuals who reside in host nation who are not citizens of the host nation or do not possess permanent resident status. Unauthorized or undocumented immigrants also include foreign-born individuals who entered the host nation legally but overstayed the authorized time period. In the United States, the term "illegal alien" is also used to refer to this group. In South Africa, the term "illegal foreigner" is also used to refer to this group.

Chapter 2

Women in Disasters

At the formative cornerstone of "Ground Zero" in our construction of structural violence, resides gender equity, bioethics of care, human capabilities, and social composition mechanisms. Structural violence, as a society or state's potential ability to fulfill an individual's needs, and the structural inequities that result in the lack of fulfillment of those needs, will be defined and explained. While social inequalities may exist in many communities, events like disasters and forced migration can markedly exacerbate pre-existing social inequities, societal ills, and medical conditions.

Not gender but gender inequity is the mechanism that places girls and women at heightened risks before, during, and after a disaster. It is acute inequities in social, political, and economic power, cultural roles, and social frameworks that trigger and ignite the firestorms of structural violence and socially constructed vulnerabilities. A homogeneous statement can be expressed on behalf of other vulnerable groups, including the economically disadvantaged, minorities (and socially marginalized), children, the elderly, the homeless, the disabled, overburdened caregivers, the mentally ill, those with chronic health issues, and so on.

The vulnerable groups of undocumented Zimbabwean and Mexican women studied in this research can be said to exist under the auspices of Giorgio Agamben's "bare life" or as "*homo sacer*"—someone who subsists or endures a life within a government's law, yet is an exile in it. Political refugees, Holocaust victims, and Guantanamo Bay's "enemy combatant" prisoners are all examples of people living in this suspended state. The "*homo sacer*" concept of the sacred (or the excluded, doomed, or accursed) man is Agamben's elucidation to an ancient Roman law: a person who banned, may be killed by anyone, yet cannot be sacrificed during a religious ritual (1995, 8). The Italian philosopher's ethico-politico stance on the "bare life" of people who are in a suspended state of "inclusive exclusion" within a government's constraints can be summed up as: ". . . the so-called sacred and inalienable rights of man prove to be completely unprotected at the very moment it is no longer possible to characterize them as rights of the citizens of a state." In his article "We Refugees," he went on to more specifically address refugees as "*homo sacer*":

> The basic point is that every time refugees no longer represent individual cases but rather a mass phenomenon . . . these organizations and the single states have proven, despite the solemn evocations of the inalienable rights of man, to be absolutely incapable not only of resolving the problem but also simply of dealing with it adequately. In this way the entire question was transferred into the hands of the police and of humanitarian organizations. (Agamben 1995, 115–16)

Much like the reanimation of people living in a state of "political statelessness" or "suspended animation"—today's contemporary politics must shake off the confusion and general aporias that characterizes modern society and its democracy, including the aporia of bare life.

Mahatma Gandhi famously referred to poverty as "the worst form of violence." Yet violence can be manifested in a myriad of forms of direct (obvious, sporadic, carried out by identifiable individual(s) for intentional harm), domestic, structural (avoidable, not always obvious, almost always invisible, can be unintentional, and carried out continuously by systematic social, political, or economic efforts, and/or embedded in institutions), and cultural—with structural violence existing as the more obscure, opaque, and indistinct form of manifested violence, oftentimes cloaked in ubiquitous practices whereby the harm is more protracted, indirect, commonplace, problematic to comprehend in scope, and provide any reparation for damages. Structural violence ensues when people are affected, injured, or impaired due to inequitable social composition (as opposed to direct and manifested physical violence Structural, or systemic, violence occurs when an institutionalized practice, scheme, or established system negatively impacts groups in an inequitable fashion, whereby people are socially, politically and/or economically exploited, oppressed, and dominated. Some examples of structural violence would include the following: elitism, ethnocentrism, classism, racism, sexism, nationalism, heterosexism, and ageism, or any other form of exploitation, poverty, denial of basic needs, or marginalization of a person. Left unchecked, structural violence frequently leads to direct violence as the oppressed and disadvantaged population(s) revolt against the institutions or governments that permit and impose these human-generated inequities in power.

The ostensible progenitor of structural violence, Johan Galtung, first coined the term "structural violence" in the 1960s. As the pioneer professor of peace and conflict research, Galtung considered the theories of structural violence and social injustice as synonymous concepts of "unequal life chances" that both usher in inequitable accesses to resources, political power, education, healthcare, or legal status. Galtung explains violence as follows: "I understand violence as the *avoidable* impairment of fundamental human needs or, to put it in more general terms, the impairment of human life, which lowers the actual degree to which someone is able to meet their needs below that which would otherwise be possible" (1993, 106). As an example, Galtung noted that if someone died from tuberculosis in the eighteenth century it would be hard to conceive of this as violence since it might have been quite unavoidable, but if he dies from it today, despite all the medical resources in the modern world, then structural violence is present (1969, 168–69). Consequently, structural violence—in all of its forms—fabricates pronounced and preventable causes of premature death, suffering, needless disabilities, as well as the exacerbation of lower acuity illnesses/diseases into higher acuity illness/disease phases. As we see from this research, the Zimbabwean and Mexican women fall victim to structural violence in that their access to lifesaving emergency medical care is obstructed, discouraged, and/or flatly denied by some xenophobic medical personnel, political posture, or institutionalized systemic procedure. And due to the avoidable, unnecessary, and preventable nature of their illnesses and treatment, their experiences are the consequence and product of structural violence.

Table 2.1 Galtung Violence Typology

	4 Need Groups			
Galtung Violence Typology	*Survival (Negation: Death)*	*Well-Being (Negation: Poverty, Illness)*	*Identity/Purpose (Negation: Alienation)*	*Freedom (Negation: oppression)*
Direct Violence	Killing	Injury, siege, poverty, sanctions	Underclass, de- or re-socialization	Repression, Imprisonment
Structural Violence	Exploitation A: Starvation or death from disease/ illness	Exploitation B: Permanent involuntary state of poverty–malnutrition and illness	Segmentation	Marginalization and Fragmentation

Johan Galtung (1969).

As we see above in Galtung's "Typology of Violence" from 1969 (Table 2.1), the "need groups" may be disadvantaged to such an extent that they starve, become terminally ill from the result of illness or disease, or die. The second category, Exploitation B, leaves the underprivileged in a constant involuntary state of poverty, usually comprising malnutrition and illness. These effects all occur within and at the culmination of multifaceted social and economic structures, and obscured legislative cycles. A noted successor of Galtung's benchmark work in structural violence, James Gilligan began a quest to look closely at the ties between structural violence and its effects on individuals' health, violent behavior, and society. As a prison psychiatrist and director of the Center for the Study of Violence at Harvard Medical School, Gilligan observed that structural violence differs from behavioral violence in three major respects: In addition to its virtual invisibility, structural violence functions more or less independently of individual behaviors; further, its problematic effects operate continuously, not just sporadically (1996). In his book *Violence: Reflections on a National Epidemic,* James Gilligan defines structural violence as "the increased rates of death and disability suffered by those who occupy the bottom rungs of society, as contrasted with the relatively lower death rates experienced by those who are above them" (1996, 192). Gilligan largely describes these "excess deaths" as "non-natural" and attributes them to the stress, shame, discrimination, and denigration that results from lower status. Gilligan paralleled the worldwide summations of structural violence to direct (armed conflict, military or political wars) violence thusly:

> Every fifteen years, on the average, as many people die because of relative poverty as would be killed in a nuclear war that caused 232 million deaths; and every single year, two to three times as many people die from poverty throughout the world as were killed by the Nazi genocide of the Jews over a six-year period. This is, in effect, the equivalent of an ongoing, unending, in fact accelerating, thermonuclear war, or genocide on the weak and poor every year of every decade, throughout the world. . . . The question as to which of the two forms of violence—structural or behavioral—is more important, dangerous, or lethal is moot, for they are inextricably related to each other, as cause to effect. (Gilligan 1996, 195–96)

When we fix and focus our view on structural violence through the lens of healthcare, we see that every country is marked by suffering, illnesses, and death, to one extent of another. But it is the distribution of the *preventable* and *manageable* illnesses and diseases in underprivileged countries that tip the scales of parity in suffering. It is these "social conditions"—these imbalances of influence—if you will, that affect and influence social justice in healthcare, and creates a poverty of lifesaving access to medication, supplies, treatment, training, and equipment to stave off human suffering from avoidable and unnecessary illness and disease. Didier Fassin in his book *Humanitarian Reason* quotes Margaret Lock concerning social sentiment on human suffering: "Efforts to reduce suffering have habitually focused on control and repair of individual bodies. The social origins of suffering and distress, including poverty and discrimination, even if fleetingly recognized, are set aside" (2012, 21).

Medical anthropologist Paul Farmer, M.D., has written several books including: *The Pathologies of Power, AIDS and Accusation: Haiti and the Geography of Blame, Haiti after the Earthquake, and Infections and Inequalities: The Modern Plagues*, all of which address structural violence and its effects on access, diagnoses, and treatment of the socioeconomically disadvantaged. Farmer describes these discriminatory social constructions as "social structures characterized by poverty and steep grades of social inequality, including racism and gender inequality" (2004, 307). Modern society, bifurcated along the impoverished and affluent lines of public status, continues to deny lifesaving and sight-saving healthcare access to the poor, oftentimes cloaked in the excuses garb of "inaccessibility," or "cost-ineffectiveness," or political jockeying for authority or celebrity, or a lack of proper funding, and so on . . . One such example of this is the disease of (standard) Tuberculosis, a malady that has been around since the time of the ancient Egyptian Pharaohs, yet access to diagnosis and a low-cost treatment developed back in 1940s remains an enduring stumbling block today in poor countries. (This example does not endeavor to include the newer strains of multidrug-resistant tuberculosis [MDR-TB], or extensively drug-resistant TB [XDR-TB], or totally drug-resistant tuberculosis [TDR-TB] forms.) Tuberculosis is a prime example of structural violence in that our modern society's current course of one six-month standard TB treatment drugs cost approximately $20—yet in 2008, there were an estimated 9.4 million new TB cases, and 1.8 million TB deaths (WHO 2010). In the same vein, issues that can make a healthy delivery and sound pregnancy risky and/or even fatal for women are, indeed, structural; so are the issues that de-value or place a nominal emphasis women's health, and limit a woman's ability and authority to seek healthcare for herself or her child(ren). In short, structural violence limits a person's life. And these limitations, with all of their physical afflictions and mental anguish, could be prevented and/or mitigated with collective civic, economic, and political demands to end social inequity.

Unlike structural violence (not caused by patient action), a patient's action must demonstrate some demonstrable level of individual responsibility, and avoid self-injurious behaviors to themselves (i.e. patient action). It is here that we should note the consequential distinction between patient factors (i.e. personal responsibility) that can lead to a patient's morbidity or mortality—versus avoidable xenophobic, discriminatory, or poor patient management factors in a clinical or hospital setting. The healthcare system can only provide equitable treatment and care if the patient participates, comprehends, and adheres to prescribed treatments, medication, early intervention in the disease, pregnancy or trauma, and follow-up care (like post-operative checks). Faulty, imprudent and/or irresponsible behavior on the patient's part leaves even the most equitable and effective healthcare system helpless and impotent. Various patient factors can include: patient delay(s) in seeking care or starting treatment; refusal to participate in physician-ordered treatment plan(s); surgical intervention or medications; continuation of destructive and/or injurious habits (such as smoking, unprotected sex, overeating, and illicit drug use); use of unqualified, unlicensed or traditional healers, midwives, etc.; cultural, superstitious, religious, familial or traditional beliefs that impede, delay or prohibit care; leaving against medical advice (signing out of hospital AMA is equal to against medical advice, which is considered one type of contributory negligence); noncompliance or the incorrect execution of doctor's orders or medication(s); injurious interference in healthcare treatment (such as a pregnant woman in antenatal program who attempts abortion or birth via relative or unlicensed healer); and/or the incorrect use of prescribed medication or the harmful use of non-prescribed medication. In the end, there must be some parameters for an individual taking personal accountability and responsibility for their own health, unless they are not capable of grasping or executing these responsibilities due to mental health or chronic/debilitating medical issues. However if the patient adheres to proper professional medical care, there can still remain a variety of avoidable factors in poor patient management in hospitals and clinics. Some of these factors would include: delay or incorrect diagnosis; transfer or referral; failure to initiate proper treatment; lack of necessary diagnostic testing; equipment and/or medication(s), staffing or supplies; understaffing (staff shortages that can lead to inadequate patient monitoring); overcrowding; a lack of basic facility needs like electricity and/or running water; poor operative techniques; lack of medical knowledge or training; dysfunctional doctor-nurse decision-making authority and communication hierarchy; and finally personal staffing factors like stress, incompetence, discrimination (xenophobia) and a lack of motivation and/or financial incentive (unpaid or low pay). Any one of these singular factors can lead directly to a patient's morbidity or mortality, and unfortunately each of these avoidable factors is usually well outside of the limits of an average patient's control. Some of these poor patient management factors directly reflect structural violence in that sub-standard facilities, equipment and staffing echo the inequitable access of training, medication, and funding to developing regions and vulnerable populations. My personal preference is to define structural violence as "macro-proportioned patterns of power" that systemically oppress and exploit individuals—causing unnecessary and continual suffering, disease and death "at the micro-individual level." To conclude our discussion of structural violence, it is of crucial consequence to again demarcate and delineate the three pivotal terms, *unnecessary, avoidable,* and *continual* when discussing a society or state's potential ability to fulfill an individual's needs and the structural inequities that result in the lack of fulfillment of those needs. As human rights activists and political science theorists, we can draw a dotted line between a state's systematic denials of emergency healthcare, as a basic human need, as a structural violation of human rights. Extreme imbalances of social power are based on structural violence, which limits individuals in their quest for equitable access to healthcare in a society. Therefore, inequity in the access to lifesaving healthcare can be regarded as tantamount to structural violence.

DISASTER TYPES AND THEIR CONSEQUENCES FOR WOMEN

While social inequalities may exist in many communities, events like forced migration markedly exacerbate pre-existing social inequities, societal ills, and medical conditions. According to Giles and Hyndman, current United Nations' High Commission for Refugees (UNHCR) policies fail to recognize "the ways in which "women" and "culture" are constructed together and in subordination," and that the diagnosis of the needs of refugee women is itself a political act, shaped by the questions asked and answers given (2004, 203). Socially constructed vulnerabilities can vary according to societal, political, and economic status and power, religion, race, gender, and most obviously, the type of the disaster event itself. In order to outline and delineate the various types of disasters, we will divide them according to the six main categories of the UN Development Programme, each with differing effects, impacts, and consequences for women. The first type of disaster we will address is the *rapid-onset disaster*, like earthquakes, and storms, that destroy homes but usually do not lead to displacement. These disasters usually leave larger major social constructions and organizations less damaged in rural expanses, but have a greater social impact on urban expanses. In the second type of disaster, the *slow-onset disaster*, like droughts and desertification, which have large social and economic impacts, but comprise greater time allowances for relocation and coping strategies. The third disaster type is the *human-induced disaster*—such as armed conflict. These conflicts may or may not cause displacement and loss of possessions, but cause more acute psychological trauma (like PTSD) than natural disasters.

As one example, in February 2009, Amnesty International drew worldwide attention to the use of rape and sexual violence as a "weapon of war" in conflicts. The controversial ad pictured a large bullet and simply stated:

Rape is cheaper than bullets. The use of sexual violence in conflicts is not a newfound concept and has been readily employed in many armed wars, but most notably and strikingly in Bosnia, the Democratic Republic of the Congo (DRC). During the 1992–1995 war in Bosnia and Herzegovina between 20,000–50,000 women were reportedly raped; in the DRC 2,200 cases of rape were reported in the first six months of 2008; only 150 of these cases came before a criminal court—and in only one case was the offender found guilty (Harvey 2009). Rape as a weapon of war can lead to a myriad of psychological, physiological, and medical crises and trauma: unwanted pregnancies, attempted self-induced abortions, infanticide, Post-Traumatic Stress Disorder (PTSD), suicide, social rejection and/or stigmatization, and life-threatening sexually transmitted diseases like HIV/AIDS. The use of "systematic rape" during times of war or conflict was recognized as a crime against humanity in 1998 via a ground-breaking decision by the ICTR and the drafting of the Rome Statute of the International Criminal Court, according to the Center for Law and Globalization at the University of Illinois (2013). One example reported by the Center was in 2001, when the International Criminal Tribunal for the former Yugoslavia convicted eight men of crimes against humanity in the case of Prosecutor vs. Kunarac, Kovac, and Vokovic, and the allegations focused exclusively on sex crimes.

A fourth category of disaster is *epidemics* (like HIV/AIDS, tuberculosis, and swine or bird flu), that can vary as either rapid or slow-onset disasters. Again, women tend to bear disproportionate caretaker burdens in epidemics or pandemics. As one example, the global HIV/AIDS pandemic is manifesting very distinct effects on women and girls, both those infected with the virus and those who lose family members to the disease. There are indications that women may become infected through sexual contact more easily than men and that they tend to become infected at a younger age (UNDP 1993, 1–2). Women also bear disproportionate burdens in caring for those who are sick with AIDS. A fifth category of disaster is *floods* that tend to cause displacement for a short time period. Lastly, the final classification of disaster, *refugee emergencies,* comprises examples such as mass persecutions, armed conflicts, and forced migration due to economic hardships, political oppression, and drug violence. These emergencies cause (by their very definition) some displacement. This type of disaster is characterized by extreme social and familial disruption, increased work demands, sexual violence, as well as psychosocial trauma. The UNHCR has given precise and noticeable responsiveness refugee women's conditions, which is echoed in an assemblage of documents, including UNHCR 1981, 1991a, 1991b, 199lc, and UNHCR and Refugee Policy Group, as well as the formation of a Senior Coordinator for Refugee Women (who is responsible to ensure that the needs and potential of refugee women are present throughout UNHCR programs) (Mocellin et al. 1994, 2). But due to the formidable variations, environments, extent, and durations of disasters and emergencies, any evaluation of "stereotypical women's challenges" in a disaster type would not only be problematical, but inaccurate. The task of providing effective and appropriate gender-aware guidance in every disaster, though, requires the active involvement of affected women.

If we focus solely on natural disasters, we see entirely new algorithms at work for gender issues. As opposed to manmade disasters, natural catastrophes, and extreme environmental events (such as hurricanes, typhoons, etc.) can introduce a distinctive set of challenges, vulnerabilities and opportunities for women. Social vulnerability is, according to Elaine Enarson, in her benchmark *Gender and Natural Disasters* book, a "function of people's relative exposure to hazard, mitigation efforts, and access to key resources needed to anticipate, cope with and recover from the effects of disastrous natural events" and that the key resources can include social power and networks, transportation, time, information, organizational skills, and literacy (2000, 16). She notes that the more socially isolated or excluded and impoverished a population may be, the less it will be able to obtain or act upon disaster warnings, take part in mitigation efforts or utilize recovery information. Enarson also noted 18 "highly vulnerable" populations of women that are at disproportionate risk in the context of natural disasters. They include women who are: undocumented; recent migrants; poor (low income); senior; head of household; indigenous; socially isolated; homeless; living alone; refugees; cognitively or physically disabled; widows; in subordinated cultural groups; caregivers with numerous dependents; subject to domestic abuse or sexual assault; chronically ill; malnourished; and those who have language barriers (2000). Clearly the Zimbabwean and Mexican women in our study would fit into several of these "highly vulnerable" classifications as undocumented and/or poor recent forced migrants and refugees from a subordinated cultural group that potentially have some form(s) of language barriers.

Within the category of forced migration as a refugee emergency, there are three primary classifications, including conflict-, disaster- and development-induced displacements (FMO 2010). While the conflict- and disaster-induced causes are widely recognized by academics and practitioners in research and aid, the lesser-known classification of development-induced includes people who are compelled to move as a result of policies and large-scale infrastructure projects such as dams, roads, ports, airports; urban clearance initiatives; mining and deforestation; and the introduction of conservation parks/reserves and biosphere projects (FMO 2010). And while forced migration and refugee emergencies affect all members and facets of familial life, for the world's women, ". . . the home is the most important place in the world, providing shelter, a space to nurture children, possible respite from violence in the streets, and for some women, the only locus of social activities" (Murray 2008, 142). Therefore women may be more disproportionately affected psychologically and physically by being forced out of their homes, separated from family, friends, and social support, and they can become more vulnerable to threats against physical security, such as abduction, rape, assault, harassment, and extortion (Murray 2008). In overcrowded refugee camps, anarchy rules, leaving unaccompanied girls and women extremely vulnerable to sexual abuse, sexual threats, and rape. Plus, in disasters and refugee scenarios, women suffer different social (menstruation taboos), psychological (more stress, trauma), and medical issues (pregnancy loss, infections), according to the WHO (2002). This research will help pinpoint and address Zimbabwean and Mexican women's "risk factors" in power, social and financial support and hardships, taboos, as well as psychological and medical issues as unrecognized refugees. These key gender-based "risk factors" in disasters and refugee emergencies expose women to greater hardships and reduce their resilience and recovery competencies.

Whereas physiological and biological differences in the sexes remain universal, social constructs of gender-based disparities in communities can change over time and vary widely. Society, culture, religion, ethics, and familial relations shape gender roles, as well as interrelated opportunities, challenges, and limitations. Feminist scholars note that: "Gender is a social construction and to specify one's gender automatically entails questions about relations of race, class and political power . . ." (Meintjes et al. 2001, 5). But gender remains at the core of most societies' organizing principals, affecting rights, responsibilities, self-efficacy, exposure to risk, and access to health care.

Many reasons contribute to socially constructed gender differences in exposure and behaviors, and the following is an abbreviated view of some of the main causes and consequences of vulnerabilities of gender risk factors in disasters worldwide (Richter 2006 and Richter 2007). I have condensed and abridged these previously published "Gender Risk Factors" into nine primary "Causes of Vulnerability" followed by four "Consequences of Vulnerability."

The first cause of vulnerability we'll address is reduced access to resources. On a global scale, women in general terms have less access to resources and less decision-making skills (one such example is illiteracy) and experiences, which are essential in disaster preparedness, mitigation, and rehabilitation (Pan American Health Organization 2004). Plus government-sponsored sex-based discrimination can render women unequal before the law, taking away women's legal authority and severely restricting women's "public life" access and participation in disaster preparedness, evacuation, mitigation training, and recovery efforts.

Second, there is a marked gendered division of labor in that women hold more underpaid jobs in agriculture, self-employment, and the informal economy sectors—sectors that are hit the hardest in natural disasters, according to the Pan American Health Organization (2004). This unbalanced gendered division of labor not only translates into women working longer hours with less social and/or economic securities than those in the informal sector, but also leaves them less able to plan for, mitigate against, and recover from natural disasters as readily as workers in the formal economy. As many as 70% of all women globally now retain positions in the informal economy, according to Enarson, and these positions in domestic service, microenterprise, and other home-based jobs put them at a heightened exposure to lose both their shelter (home) and economic resources in disasters (2000). In most countries, according to the World Bank, women are less likely than men to participate in the formal labor economic market—meaning that they are not only less likely to be employed, but also to be actively seeking a job (2012). The same report noted that women are more likely to participate in "vulnerable jobs" (like unpaid family work and self-employment) in the South Asia and Middle East and North Africa regions, with a gender gap between men and men in these "vulnerable jobs" ranging from 8% to 15%. Nussbaum reported that on average, women's rates of employment participation are about 50% that of men, with lower rates in South Asia at 29% and in Arab states only 16% (2005). For the auspices of this study, the four countries researched in this literature reflect varying percentages of women employed in non-agricultural jobs: 39% in Mexico, 45% in South Africa, 48% in the U.S.A., and 22% in Zimbabwe, according to current World Bank's Gender and Equality Statistics website (2013).

The third consequence of vulnerability is the constraint of female social taboos, restrictions, and isolation. Globally women can suffer from less personal autonomy, as well as a lack of knowledge of how to access emergency assistance, and/or the capacity to do so. But particularly in disasters, women suffer different social taboos (menstruation, head cover, and nudity), psychological issues (lower value status for help, more stress, higher rates of PTSD), patriarchal/religious/cultural restrictions (female receipt of medical care from male-only healthcare provider, loss of head and body covering) (WHO 2002). For example, in the aftermath of the 2005 Hurricane Katrina, high rates of mental illness and parenting stress were observed in female survivors resulting in serious implications for the mental health of children (WHO 2002).

Fourth, women in general hold a decreased ability to migrate for employment and aid. Due to home, child, and/or elderly care issues, women are less able to migrate for employment (Enarson 2003). Plus, in certain countries there may be transportation, employment, and travel restrictions regarding women that do not allow them to make or act on employment decisions without direct familial and/or patriarchal consent. A study by the World Health

Organization (WHO) and UNICEF Joint Monitoring Programme estimated that 200 million hours are spent each and every day globally—just in the activity of collecting water (2010). The same study noted that in surveys from 45 developing countries women and children shoulder the vast majority of chores involved in collecting water in the preponderance of households. Just this singular task can keep women from time spent at an income-generating job, in education, etc.

The fifth consequence of vulnerability is that women, in general, are the most likely person to be/become sole economic providers for family members. Following a disaster, a woman is more likely to be/become sole economic providers in post-displacement scenarios for dependent family members such as grandparents, disabled relatives, ill family members, and children. This is sometimes referred to as the post-disaster "flight of men," which is a well-documented phenomenon recorded in Bangladesh cyclones, the 1949 Malawi drought, and Hurricane Mitch in Central America. Additionally, researchers and relief workers noted the redirecting of relief assets by men from their family to additional "outsider" households was reported in Miami after Hurricane Andrew (Delaney and Shrader 2000). That same report noted that one year after Hurricane Andrew, 50% of Honduran and 40% of Nicaraguan households were maintained solely by women.

As a sixth basis of vulnerability, we will cite women's disproportionate access, pre-existing issues and conditions, and treatment in healthcare. Due to inadequate or non-existent obstetrics/gynecological healthcare, female physicians and limited reproductive control, women suffer from limited healthcare access, infections, premature births, malnutrition, unwanted pregnancies, and pregnancy losses (WHO 2002). As one example, in the 2004 southeastern Asian Tsunami, the WHO reported some 80% of the total fatalities in Indonesia and Sri Lanka were women. "Due to their reproductive roles, women are particularly negatively affected if the basic healthcare infrastructure is severely damaged or health expenditures are reduced to re-allocate funds for immediate disaster response purposes" (Neumayer 2007). Additionally, women who have undergone female genital mutilation, also known as female circumcision, are at extremely high risk for complications like caesarean section (surgical intervention) delivery, postpartum hemorrhage, and prolonged hospitalization. Not surprisingly, complications increased in a direct and corresponding manner to the level of severity of the type of genital mutilation. As classified by the WHO system, there are four types: Type I (removal of the prepuce and/or clitoris), Type II (removal of clitoris and labia minora), Type III (removal of part or all of the external genitalia with stitching or narrowing of the vaginal opening, also known as infibulation), and Type IV (any harmful procedures to the female genitalia for non-medical purposes, like pricking, piercing, incising, scraping, and/or cauterization). Women who had undergone the most dangerous form of genital mutilation (Type III) bore a 30% increased risk for delivery by surgical C-section and a 70% greater risk of postpartum hemorrhage than women had not had any genital mutilation, according to the WHO (2008). In infibulation and severe excision, defibulation (re-cutting of vaginal opening) must be performed during childbirth, needlessly exposing women to a litany of fetal and/or maternal complications such as obstructed labor, perineal tears, infection, hypovolemic shock, neonatal mortality, vesicovaginal or rectovaginal fistulae (holes that permit urine and feces to seep into the vagina), and damage to the anal sphincter. Any deficiencies or absence of female healthcare supplies and gender-aware services can place women at higher risk for illness, increase morbidity and/or mortality rates, and/or increase other long-term medical interventions such as multiple emergency room, physician, and therapist visits. As for comprehensive maternal mortality ratios (the number of women who die during pregnancy and childbirth—per 100,000 live births) in the four countries in this study are as follows: 50 in Mexico, 300 in South Africa, 21 in the U.S.A., and 570 in Zimbabwe, according to the World Bank's Gender and Equality Statistics website (2013).

Seventh cause of vulnerability is the general lack of gender-disaggregated data in census studies, disaster research, employment, social sciences studies, and other areas. According to the World Bank (2007), one of the primary reasons it has been so difficult for non-governmental charities and government agencies to pin down women's specific needs in manmade and natural disasters is the dearth of gender-disaggregated data. There are no gender-specific data on mortalities in 90% of developing nations, on unemployment in 75% of the global population, and half of the world lives in places where economic activity by gender has not been reported for at least the last decade (WHO 2007). "The fact that we still have not fully mainstreamed gender issues amounts to the exclusion of women. For data that is fundamental to promote growth and poverty reduction, we need to make women more visible in statistics," says Maya Buvinic, director of gender and development for the World Bank's Poverty Reduction and Economic Management Network (World Bank 2007, 1). Raymond Weist of the U.N. Development Programme concurs with Buvinic's views, and notes that a lack of gender focus or "gender blindness" can be a probable, perhaps even predictable, shortfall in research (1994, 6–8). He adds that there is "no reason to expect disaster-related research to be less gender-biased than social research in general," and that the study of the needs of women is "not to extricate them from their social systems," but for models of disaster management to be "linked to development theory and integrated with theories of behavior that embody cultural rules and social contexts as well as global political and economic processes" (Weist et al. 1994, 6–8). Currently there are two primary sources of global gender-disaggregated data, the United Nation Development Programme's Gender-related Development Index and the United Nation Development Programme's Gender Empowerment Measure (GEM) report. According to UNDP, the Gender-related Development Index (GDI), measures achievement in the much the same way their Human Development Index (HDI) does, but it also measures inequalities in achievement between women and men. The methodology "imposes a penalty for inequality, such that the GDI falls when the achievement levels of both women and men in a country go down or when the disparity between their achievements increases" (UNDP 1). So, the greater the gender disparity, the lower a country's GDI is when compared with its HDI. According to the latest GDI report for 2007–2008, the four countries' value and global ranking among 171 countries are as follows: U.S.A. (0.937, 12th in global ranking), Mexico (0.820, 52nd in global ranking), South Africa (0.667, 121st in global ranking), and Zimbabwe (0.505, 151st in global ranking), showing that women in both the U.S.A. and South Africa enjoy more gender equality than their corresponding refugee counterpart countries, Mexico and Zimbabwe (UNDP 2007). The second measure, GEM, is a measure of agency, evaluating progress in advancing women's standing in political and economic forums, and examines the extent to which women and men are able to actively participate in economic and political life and take part in decision making. So, while the GDI focuses on each country's expansion of capabilities, the GEM is concerned with the actual, day-to-day implementation of those capabilities. According to the latest GEM report of 2007–2008, there are only two nations among the four discussed that were ranked and valued: U.S.A. and Mexico, with the GEM ranking U.S.A. at 15th worldwide with 0.762, and Mexico as the 46th worldwide with 0.589 (UNDP 2007). UNDP values for GEM rankings for South Africa and Zimbabwe were unavailable at the time of publication.

As an eighth cause of vulnerability, women's underrepresentation and/or subordinate representation in high-level emergency management organizations and decision-making roles leaves women less visible in the mainstream's "malestream" processes. Some of the more ancillary obstacles to women's effective involvement and input in the political arena are their conspicuous underrepresentation in governmental "decision-maker" positions. Though women have long been witnessed as keen social monitors, local community organizers, and strong informal leaders in their communities—women made up only 10% of the world's parliamentary representatives and less than 4% of cabinet officials by 1980 (Nussbaum 2005). Considering the four countries we are particularly studying, the proportion of seats held by women in national parliaments in Mexico is 26%, in South Africa is 42%, in the U.S.A. is 17%, and in Zimbabwe is 15%, according to the World Bank's Gender and Equality Statistics website (2013).

The final and ninth factor we will address is the increase in women's domestic and economic chores/burdens in their post-disaster homes or shelters. Inadequate refugee shelters (for cooking, bathing, etc.) can leave women even less time, freedom and mobility to look for work, according to the Pan American Health Organization (2004).

Now that we've listed nine causes of women's social constructions of vulnerability in disasters, we'll address four of the major consequences of vulnerability. These consequences can be viewed as the after-effects of structural violence, combined with gender discrimination and gender-based inequity. The first consequence is a woman's loss of her household "bargaining position." When a woman's economic resources are taken away, her "bargaining position" in the household is adversely affected, according to the Pan American Health Organization (2004). A second consequence of vulnerability is a women's heightened perception of risk. In general, studies find that women are more safety conscious, risk averse, and perceive disaster threats as more serious and risky than men. Studies show that girls and women suffer more distress and emotional disorders in disasters, though overall declines in emotional well-being may be due to expanded caregiving roles (WHO 2002). Some studies have led to the speculative inference that women are more fearful in general due to their greater vulnerability to crime, and physical and sexual violence in perilous environments (like post-disaster settings, refugee camps, and shelters). In a predominance of studies, men were found (in general) to engage in more risky behaviors than women and women's higher perceived likelihood of negative outcomes and lower expectation of enjoyment somewhat interceded in reduced inclinations toward risks in gambling, recreation, and health domains (Glaser et al. 2006). This gender difference was due to, in part, women's more optimistic beliefs of the probability of good outcomes. A meta-analysis by Byrnes, Miller, and Schafer (1999) studied over 150 papers on gender differences in risk perception, and the authors concluded that the research "clearly" indicated that "male participants are more likely to take risks than female participants," with males identifying less risk than women and a greater probability of engaging in risk-taking behaviors (Byrnes et al. 1999, 377). Since studies do hold out that men and women differ in their perception of risk, the assessments in the probability and severity of negative outcomes, it is a plausible and even probable hypothesis that the sexes would then also differ in their reactions, attentiveness to warnings, and preparedness in disasters. Disaster researchers should strive to actively exploit these gender differences in their evacuation communications and their family disaster preparedness promotions.

Perhaps the most widely known, researched, and publicized consequence to vulnerability is the sharp uptick in domestic and sexual violence during and after disasters. In the wake of the loss of social authority (such as a police force), women are left less protected from crimes like rape, violence, theft, and other forms of exploitation in refugee and post-disaster settings. As one example, a 2007 survey of displaced Hurricane Katrina residents living in trailers found that nearly half of those surveyed reported being in worse health than the day before Hurricane Katrina, 30 per cent had been victims of theft, and one in six women reported being a victim of domestic violence (Whoriskey 2007). Domestic and sexual violence against women is a social reality that impacts a women's vulnerability during and after a disaster. According to noted gender and disaster expert Elaine Enarson's "Violence against Women in Disasters" research: "Women in violent relationships are a vulnerable population less visibly at risk than poor women, refugees, single mothers, widows, senior or disabled women" and impacts an estimated one in four women in the U.S.A. and Canada, and as much as 60% of women in Africa, Latin America, and Asia (2006, 1). Disaster planners and providers should take proactive steps to prevent and discourage GBV by requiring good lighting around toilets and shelters, and organizing public events in the daytime to promote safety, and encouraging women to travel only in groups (and never unaccompanied) in disaster-affected areas.

The final consequence is women's more direct and higher dependence on public and social services. These public and social services and facilities can include schools, clinics, child care centers, public services, as well as water, fuel (wood), crops and other natural resources. Women, in general, are more connected to their children's school system and education, and more likely than men to manage and use natural resources on a daily basis (Enarson 2003).

These aforementioned risk factors that can be considered the more simply identified "low-hanging fruit" in gender-based disaster and refugee research. But while significant disparities emerge when we view female healthcare through the lens of justice, disaster aid, human rights and gender discrimination, it begs the question what is gender equity? And how do societies and governments begin to determine, measure, and design a system in which to equitably allocate those resources? The processes of the public planning of the formulation and fulfillment of its citizen's needs will be addressed subsequently.

Indeed, it may prove a simpler task to evaluate, study, and quantify gender needs than to attempt to distribute, even somewhat equitably, finite resources and political, social, and fiscal power throughout a society in a "gender-equitable" manner. The (in itself) presumptuous declaration of "equitable" distribution assumes that equitable—as in impartial, reasonable, just, rightful, and fair—allocation of assets, income, and resources has occurred, or could ever occur. But what is "equitable" and to whom? And equality based on what internal traits or external situations like age, gender, abilities or disabilities, environmental or economic dilemmas, or a predisposition to illnesses? In Amartya Sen's landmark book *Inequality Reexamined*, the author has this to say about the (seemingly) impartial and objective parity when debating the formidable idiom of the "equality of man":

> The powerful rhetoric of "equality of man" often tends to deflect attention away from these differences. Even though such rhetoric (e.g. "all men are born equal") is typically taken to be part and parcel of egalitarianism, the effect of ignoring the interpersonal variations can, in fact, be deeply inegalitarian, in hiding the fact that equal consideration for all may demand very unequal treatment in favor of the disadvantaged. (Sen 1992, 1)

If we can resolutely declare anything about humanity with unequivocal certainty, it is that human diversity is a fundamental cornerstone in the building of conceptual social equality. Human diversity and disparate equalities, according to Sen, exist not just in theory, but actuality, in that our internal characteristics (age, gender, abilities, talents, predisposition to illness, etc.) and external circumstances (fiscal assets, societal backgrounds, environmental circumstances, etc.) vary extensively. "It is precisely because of such diversity that the insistence on egalitarianism in one field requires the rejection of egalitarianism in another," wrote Sen (1992, p. xi). The author also argues that the John Rawls, or the Rawlsian theory of "justice as fairness," doesn't go far enough to neither give credit nor responsibility to a person who has no control over distinct circumstances, such as having poor or rich parents, or lacking a set of natural talents. Sen again stresses that people should be viewed through the lens of their freedom to achieve rather than their actual achievements. Martha Nussbaum concurs with Sen that the Rawlsian approach does not do enough to show how resources can (or cannot) facilitate function. Like the difference between starving (life constrained) and fasting (life chosen), individuals should enjoy the right and freedom to choose whether or not to utilize their capabilities. Nussbaum also reported there are three different types of capabilities (basic, internal, and combined) and that "the aim of public policy is the production of combined capabilities," which are "internal capabilities combined with suitable external conditions for the exercise of the function" (2005, 313). It is here we see the emphasis on the quality of life, rather the more liberal, or even socialistic, approach of a single-minded approach to quantity (as in the egalitarian distribution of resources).

At its worst, gender equity pigeonholes women as helpless and hapless victims, tossed about by the caprice of uncompassionate governments and evil men. Gender equity should never seek to become a divisive zero-sum game, in which every word written on female suffering leads to one less word written on male suffering, or vice versa. And certainly gender equity should never seek to condone nor suggest that men remain unaffected by disasters, emergency healthcare issues, and emergencies, instead it should serve as a filtered "gender lens" that illustrates how men and women are constrained by their socialization and disproportionately impacted by disasters.

At its best, gender equity should seek to highlight and uncover sex- and gender-based differences that might be more effectively harnessed in disaster planning, mitigation, response, emergency healthcare services, and recovery efforts, where women take on roles as capable citizens with gender-specific aptitudes, skilled community competencies, and leadership abilities. Gender equity, concurring with Amartya Sen, aims for women's capability and freedom to fairly and legitimately reach their own personal and functional capabilities. This pragmatic approach translates into freedom from oppression, and an enforced (not merely theoretical, but applied) zero tolerance policy for any political, social, or religious subversion or limitations placed on those conferred freedoms.

ARE WOMEN HUMAN?

Since the 1900s, there have been many international accords and declarations testifying to women's equitable nature under human rights laws (Table 2.2). In 1945, the United Nations established the elimination of any gender-based discrimination, and in 1948 the Universal Declaration of Human Rights abolished any "laws, customs, regulations and practices that are discriminatory to women" (Article 2). In 1979 an international legal instrument—the Convention on the Elimination of all Discrimination against Women (CEDAW—also known as the Treaty for the Rights of Women) was adopted by the UN General Assembly, and as of January 2013, 185 countries had ratified CEDAW. The convention contains a preamble and 30 articles and sets out to not only create what a definition for discrimination against women, but also plans of action, reporting mechanisms and enforcement of the treaty. The Convention on the Elimination of all Discrimination against Women of 1979 defines discrimination against women as follows:

> For the purposes of the present Convention, the term "discrimination against women" shall mean any distinction, exclusion or restriction made on the basis of sex which has the effect or purpose of impairing or nullifying the recognition, enjoyment or exercise by women, irrespective of their marital status, on a basis of equality of men and women, of human rights and fundamental freedoms in the political, economic, social, cultural, civil or any other field (CEDAW, Article 1).

When a country chooses to adopt CEDAW, they commit to endorse and maintain several key precepts, including (but not limited to) the incorporation, establishment and pledge to uphold equity in their legal system (via the abolition of discriminatory laws and adoption of legislation that prohibit discrimination); protection of women against discrimination in public institutions; and to eliminate discrimination by people, organizations, or businesses. According to the United Nations WOMEN (United Nations Entity for Gender Equality and the Empowerment of Women, Division for the Advancement of Women in the Department of Social and Economic Affairs), CEDAW provides the basis for realizing equality between women and men through ensuring women's equal access to, and equal opportunities in, political and public life—including the right to vote and to stand for election—as well as education, health, and employment (UN WOMEN 2013). CEDAW is the only international human rights treaty that upholds women's reproductive rights, as well as a woman's right to obtain, alter, and keep their nationality and the nationality of their children. Countries that ratify CEDAW also agree to combat the trafficking and exploitation of women, turn in a national report at least every four years, and to account for any actions they have taken to observe CEDAW's obligations.

The United States is among a small minority of countries that have not yet ratified CEDAW, along with other nations like Afghanistan, Iran, and Sudan. The United States has the controversial distinction of being the only country in the Western Hemisphere and the only industrialized democracy that has not ratified this treaty. As of March 2013, the U.S.A. had not ratified CEDAW. According to Amnesty International, "The principles espoused in the Treaty for the Rights of Women are consistent with those in U.S. laws. . . . The Treaty would nonetheless help efforts to enhance U.S. laws with respect to violence against women, access to legal protections, and other human rights. Lack of U.S. ratification serves as a disincentive for governments to uphold CEDAW's mandate and their obligations under it to end discrimination against women. With U.S. ratification, the Women's Convention would become a much stronger instrument in support of women's struggles to achieve full protection and realization of their rights" (2009). South Africa ratified CEDAW in December 1995, as well as the Optional Protocol in 2005. South Africa ratified the "Protocol to the African Charter on Human and Peoples' Rights on the Rights of Women in Africa" in 2005. The Women in Law & Development (WiLDAF—West Africa) in Lome, Togo, distributes a "simplified" version of the Protocol to the African Charter on Human and People's Rights (ACHPR) on the Rights of Women in Africa. This simplified version utilizes several streamlined drawings to assist, educate, and raise awareness of women's rights. This simplified version of the Protocol should be a great and effective tool for women's organizations working at the grassroots level with semi-literate, illiterate, and non-English speaking rural

Table 2.2 Gender Instruments Timeline, RSA and U.S.A.

Selected Key South African and American Gender and Human Rights Instruments
Universal Declaration of Human Rights (1948) declared that: "Everyone has the right to a standard of living adequate for the health and well-being of oneself and one's family, including food, clothing, housing, and medical care," and abolished any "laws, customs, regulations and practices that are discriminatory to women." (Article 2).
In U.S.A.: federal Equal Pay Act (1963), Civil Rights Act (1964), and Education Amendments (Title VII and IX) in the 1970s.
Convention on the Elimination of all Discrimination against Women (CEDAW) (1979): defined discrimination against women (Article 1), and introduced plans of action, reporting mechanisms and enforcement measures of this international legal instrument. South Africa ratified CEDAW in December 1995 and the Optional Protocol in 2005. As of 2013, the U.S.A. has not ratified.
☑ *South Africa* ☒ *U.S.A.*
Mexico (1975)—1st world conference on status of women coincided with "International Women's Year"—United Nations General Assembly identified three key objectives that would become the basis for the work of the United Nations on behalf of women: (1) full gender equality and the elimination of gender discrimination; (2) the integration and full participation of women in development and (3) an increased contribution by women in the strengthening of world peace.
UNHCR (1991) Guidelines on the Protection of Refugee Women U.N. Doc. ES/SCP/67. More guidelines from UNHCR in 2002: Guidelines on International Protection: Gender-related persecution within the context of Article 1A(2) of the 1951 Convention, and 1967 Protocol relating to the Status of Refugees, UN Doc. HCR/GIP/02/01.
In South Africa: Constitution of the Republic of South Africa (1995): guarantees equality and freedom from discrimination (section 9).
Beijing (1995): provided a "Plan for Action" and introduced "gender mainstreaming."
Declaration on the Elimination of Violence against Women (1993)—was 1st international human rights instrument to exclusively and explicitly address the issue of violence against women in that it violates, impairs or nullifies women's human rights and their exercise of freedoms. It defined gender-based abuse as "any act of gender-based violence that results in, or is likely to result in, physical, sexual or psychological harm or suffering to women, including threats of such acts, coercion or arbitrary deprivation of liberty, whether occurring in public or in private life." A/RES/48/104.
In South Africa: Gender Guidelines for Asylum Determination (1999)—accepted these guidelines suggested by the National Consortium on Refugee Affairs (an NGO).
Resolution 1325 (October 2000) UN Security Council—mandate to ensure women's voices are heard during peace-building efforts.
The Protocol to the African Charter on Human and Peoples' Rights on the Rights of Women in Africa (2005), also known as the Maputo Protocol, was adopted by the African Union on July 11, 2003 and was in force on November 25, 2005.

and urban populations. Other tools like global conferences, such as 2005s "Beijing Plus Ten," attempt to empower and improve the lives of women by establishing a guide for national governments to set public policy. The conference's Platform for Action (PFA) provided benchmarks for citizens to measure their governments' implementation of the Beijing commitments and spelled out specific human rights. Some global mandates, like the UNHCR's *Guidelines on the Protection of Refugee Women,* have directly addressed women's unique healthcare issues by recommending a "high priority to the provision of primary healthcare, including maternal and child health services, gynecological services, birthing care, counseling regarding sexually transmitted diseases, family planning programs, and health education regarding harmful practices such as female circumcision" (1991).

Bridging women's personal needs and roles within political constructs and frameworks are Maxine Molyneaux and Caroline Moser, two pivotal feminist theoreticians that helped form "strategic gender interests" concepts into transformative practical global feminist applications. Their theoretical development of practical gender needs and gender roles in humanitarian interventions and disasters is a pivotal aspect of this research's standpoint and theories. The term "strategic gender needs" was first coined by Maxine Molyneaux in 1985. Molyneaux's work in strategic gender needs assisted in developing gender planning and policy development tools like the Moser Framework, a "planning methodology aimed at the emancipation of women from their subordination and their achievement of equality, equity and empowerment . . . related to gender in development interventions at all levels, including policy, program, project, or community work" (PSIA 2012, 1). Strategic gender interests refer to interventions that tackle fundamental issues related to women's subordination and/or gender inequities. Strategic gender interests are long term, generally not based on material goods, and are often associated to status, power, and/or equity (structural) transformations in society, such as equal-rights legislation, reproductive choice, and increased participation in (political, economic, and social) decision-making functions.

The Moser Gender Planning Framework, utilized by the World Bank and International Labour Organization, was developed by Caroline Moser in 1993. The "Moser Framework" introduces the idea of a woman's so-called "triple role" (over a 24-hour period) as a productive (tasks that are monetarily reimbursed), reproductive (tasks associated with child rearing/raising and caretaking of the home like cooking, cleaning), and community involvement (tasks related to collective support and community gain) (Moser 1993). And perhaps even more importantly, the Moser Gender Planning Framework clearly distinguishes, evaluates, and measures practical needs (immediate needs necessary to ensure safety, heath, and basic needs, such as water, sanitation, healthcare, etc., that do not necessarily transform gender discriminatory power structures) from strategic needs (that advance women's equity and empowerment by challenging power structures like laws, domestic violence, etc.)—a central point of distinction in the formation of both Molyneaux's and Moser's standpoints and feminist theories (Moser 1993). Moser explains that policy approaches to low-income Third-World women "have shifted, mirroring shifts in macro-economic development policies" (1993). Moser's work also identifies five policy needs approaches which include: welfare (1950–1970s) where women are viewed as passive beneficiaries of development; equity (1st Women In Development (WID) approach, 1976–1985) women are seen as active participants in development, the triple-role of women is acknowledged, and women's subordinate position is challenged; anti-poverty (2nd WID approach, a "milder" version of equity, 1970s) women's poverty is seen as a problem of underdevelopment, not of subordination and recognizes the productive role of women; efficiency (3rd WID approach, 1980s) focuses on women's economic contribution and capacity to compensate for declining social services; and finally, empowerment (most recent approach) greater self-reliance is mandated, and women's subordination is owed to not only male oppression but also colonial and neo-colonial oppression (International Labour Organization 2013). All of these five approaches have, or have had in the past, varying degrees of acceptance by NGOs and governments, primarily to the policies' avoidance or criticism of Western feminism, challenges to social order/power, self-sufficiency (or lack thereof), or direct contestations with political/social and/or economic directives.

Charters like the Moser Gender Planning Framework and other mandates that define and enforce gender and/or human rights can be defined, implemented, and enforced by a variety of authorities, including governments, NGOs, and international humanitarian agencies such as the UNHCR. But according to Douzinas, "Governments are the enemy against whom human rights were conceived as a defense" (2003, 161). He argues that the business of government is to govern and *not* follow moral principles, so the institutions themselves can find themselves at odds with internally or externally mandated human rights accords. Douzinas states that the government-operated international human rights law is the best illustration of the "poacher turned gamekeeper" (2003, 161). Clearly in times of national crises (such as the forced Zimbabwean migration into South Africa and the mass migration of unrecognized Mexicans into the U.S.A.), governments can be deeply conflicted and inconsistent in their assumed roles as an impartial and "fair" assessor, enforcer, and provider of humanitarian services. Campbell concurs with Douzina's assessment in that the cherished values of impartiality and neutrality (which allows NGOs and humanitarian agencies and efforts to be seen as "apolitical" or "nonpolitical") is very tenuous in times of crises, so aid roles must be clearly defined in the way that international humanitarian law grants rights to individuals and gives duties to states (1998). Additionally, these laws must confront and define the parameters of how these rights are to be accorded to individuals, and for women oftentimes these rights are linked to maternal or familial relationships rather than individual human rights—which we will now examine forthwith.

MORE THAN A UTERUS: MATERNAL CARE ETHICS

When we look to Agamben's *Sovereign Power and Bare Life*, an account from 1998 on the politics of the sovereignty in the West, the emblem of modern sovereign power, the *homo sacer*, is a male. But if we take an in-depth look at today's forced migration crises among Mexican and Zimbabwean populations, we see human rights violations and arenas of healthcare emergencies as most widely portrayed and recognized with a female face. As Edkins notes, the person of the female "would seem to be foundational in the figuration of the humanitarian international and the extension of the sovereignty of the West" (2000, 20).

Sara Ruddick, long considered the original female forerunner of the theory of maternal care ethic methodology, wrote the article "Maternal Thinking" in 1980, what is counted as a pioneer articulation of a feminist ethics of care approach. She employs mothering (either from a man or woman) as the basis from which she classifies maternal attitudes, capabilities and virtues, including the concepts of "preservative love" (preserving the life of a child, a work of protection); "attentive love" (unselfish attention and reflectivity); fostering growth, and training for social acceptability (socialization). Ruddick's approach to care ethics assisted creating the foundation of feminist politics of peace, but also gave rise to the conceptualization of the importance of morality and virtue in care ethics overall. Ruddick, Nussbaum, and Virginia Held all employed maternal standpoints (to both women and men) and perspectives to develop care ethics via moral (virtuous), social, and political theories.

Yet in any type of aid, women's right to care should be based on individual human rights—rather than on some familial, child-caring, or maternal-based relationships ("women and their dependent children")—which are often considered as core organizational classifications in aid, refugee, and disaster programs. Women bear disproportionate caregiver responsibilities, and their predicaments in disasters and emergencies are coupled indissolubly (and oftentimes indistinguishably) to their offspring and their dependent family members. Giles and Hyndman write that while women are encumbered by their gendered responsibilities, and in disasters and relief they are often referred to as a singular entity: "*womenandchildren*"—a term which "essentializes the maternal relationship," and connotes that women "deserve to be helped" (2004, 203). In a thought-provoking and curious gender-bending twist, men are not usually identified as a parent or defined by their household duties. This problematic, gendered attitude plays into the "essentialist construct," state Giles and Hyndman, an attitude that does nothing to elevate women's status, but in fact, perpetuates the myth that women are ineffectual victims, forever encumbered by their gendered responsibilities (2004, 203). This is a view supported by feminist theorist Catherine MacKinnon, the author of the book aptly titled *Are Women Human?* that addresses "the social, legal, religious and political orthodoxies which continue to condone the rape, genital mutilation, slavery, economic impoverishment, imposed illiteracy and oppression of women worldwide" (2006, i). This research, along with feminist theorists like MacKinnon, Held, Tronto, Nussbaum, and others, continues to question why women continue to be deprived of basic human rights—like healthcare, literacy, self efficacy, political liberation and participation, respect, and employment—and be denied full human status and fair quality of life in social reality. This research will help pinpoint and address both perceived and real obstacles in Zimbabwean and Mexican women's social power, rights, and self-efficacy in obtaining healthcare as unrecognized refugees.

But when we address gender equity, there is an urgent need to uncover and condemn any system and/or social/political/religious policies that seek to bypass, mute or oppress women. According to Human Rights Watch: "Cultural relativism, which argues that there are no universal human rights and that rights are culture-specific and culturally determined, is still a formidable and corrosive challenge to women's rights to equality and dignity in all facets of their lives. . . . Arguments that sustain and excuse these human rights abuses—those of cultural norms, "appropriate" rights for women, or western imperialism—barely disguise their true meaning: that women's lives matter less than men's" (2007, 12).

In conclusion, it is of crucial consequence to emphasize and stress the terms *unnecessary, avoidable,* and *continual* when discoursing a society or state's potential ability to fulfill an individual's needs and the structural inequities that result in the lack of fulfillment of those needs. As human rights activists and political science theorists, we can draw a discernible thread between a state's systematic denials of emergency healthcare, as a basic human need, as a structural violation of human rights. Extreme imbalances of social power are based on structural violence, and therefore inequity in the access to lifesaving healthcare can be regarded as tantamount to structural violence. Through our discussion in this chapter's research, it is clear that women have unique and gender-distinctive physical, psychological, social, and economic needs, vulnerabilities, capabilities and opportunities in disasters. Perhaps even more importantly, women are an overlooked and often underutilized, but vital part of disaster mitigation and response efforts, whether they act in their traditional roles or transcend them.

There remains a tremendous global need to fight against the dehumanization and marginalization of women in disaster aid and refugee programs. It may only be through the worldwide promotion of women's rights (based on universal human rights, and state-sponsored and enforced laws) that true equity in development and assistance might be realized. This is a fight for women to be fully and completely human and equal, which will require heroic unity and solidarity in order to end timeworn social and political and economic traditions, practices and laws that continue to oppress women. Ultimately, the struggle for undocumented Zimbabwean and Mexican women's human rights and equity must be about stopping discrimination and violence against women, making women's lives count (equally) to men's—and to unleash the wonderfully vast, but as yet untapped, human potential of women to successfully participate as strategic leaders in social, political, fiscal and global development.

Chapter 3

Asylum and Immigration

The Statue of Liberty at Ellis Island, New York, in the United States welcomes migrants and visitors to its golden shores with the following compassionate and benevolent soliloquy:

Give me your tired, your poor,
Your huddled masses yearning to breathe free,
The wretched refuse of your teeming shore,
Send these, the homeless, tempest-tost to me,
I lift my lamp beside the golden door!

—Emma Lazarus, "The New Colossus," 1883

But if South Africa had a corresponding counterpart to the Statue of Liberty inviting in the "tired, weak, and oppressed"—it would be facing Zimbabwe. The United States and South Africa have both tentatively teetered between dizzying epochs of worldwide refuge-haven claims and exploding immigrant strains as two of the world's top asylum destinations. And like the United States, South Africa has adopted a "quiet diplomacy" foreign policy stance, if you will, toward President Mugabe's millions of "economic migrants" and political refugees. Therefore, the vast majorities of these Zimbabweans are deemed illegal and subject to deportation. Furthermore, some South Africans have grown to resent the long-term encroachment of these undocumented Zimbabwean migrants into their struggling labor markets, exposing them and making them vulnerable to violent clashes like the xenophobic attacks that killed 60 foreign immigrants (that included and targeted many Zimbabweans) in 2008, then reignited as xenophobic violence during the 2010 international soccer World Cup, and then again in 2015's attacks that killed 7 and displaced thousands.

In an analogous and markedly paradigmatic parallelism, like South Africa, the United States has adopted a rather lethargic "quiet diplomacy" foreign policy toward the violent Mexican drug cartels' massacres and the long-term exodus of undocumented Mexican "economic migrants" into the United States. Therefore, the vast majorities of these Mexicans are deemed illegal in the U.S.A. and are subject to deportation. Furthermore, some Americans have grown to resent the long-term encroachment of these undocumented Mexican migrants into their already stressed labor markets. But this xenophobic stance can make Mexican migrants vulnerable to extortion, violence, theft, and even death. The bloodiest example of this was the August 2010 massacre of 72 Mexicans who were attempting to cross the U.S./Texas border (*USA Today*). According to the newspaper report, the lone survivor of the attack identified the killers as drug cartel members who forced the human trafficker/smuggler to give up his "migrant cargo" so the drug gang could kidnap them and hold them as ransom to their U.S.-based family members.

These comparable and doppelganger-counterparts of South African and American crises can both fundamentally be interpreted as failed foreign policies to acknowledge political, economic, and social crises across and inside the host country's borders—coupled with a conspicuous indifference to migrants' exploitation, treatment, and protection. Dealing with the aftermath of these xenophobic attacks and violent massacres has become a daunting political gambol and a social to-and-fro swing in order to (even somewhat) safely circumvent immigration "landmines" for South African and United States citizens and their elected officials. Both countries have made both minor and major attempts to prosecute attackers, process migrants and refugee claims, protect migrants from exploitation, implement political "damage control," as well as enact a variety of political and social "soul-searching" endeavors via adjustments in legislation, administration, dispensation, and enforcement policies.

But countries like the U.S.A., Canada, and Australia have (literally) been built on human migration. Migration, whether so-called voluntary or forced, is fraught with difficulties. It involves uprooting families, leaving friends, and breaking the social customs and values that have provided a sense of continuity and self. People who are smuggled or cross borders clandestinely can be placed in situations that threaten the physical and psychological health of the migrant. In today's world, modern-day migration is less structured than in the previous decades and there has been a palpable hardening of attitudes and policies on migration, and all the while undocumented migrants face more precarious health and social environments.

While this research does not attempt to study healthcare access in host nations among recognized refugees or (foreign-born) naturalized citizens, it seeks to study only female migrants that are considered undocumented, forced, or illegal immigrants without legal migration status in either South Africa (Zimbabwean migrants) or the U.S.A. (Mexican migrants) who have sought out emergency healthcare. Therefore there is a need to address specific international, regional, and/or national laws and treatises that address rights to asylum and healthcare access to these particular groups of undocumented women. In this chapter, several undocumented migrants' issues will be addressed, including: local (state), regional, federal, and international asylum and immigration treatises pertaining to South Africa and the United States; the constructive (positive vibrant labor force and cultural enrichment) and negative (human trafficking, labor exploitation, and healthcare and federal/state aid abuses) "pushes" and "pulls" of migration in host countries; policy enforcement and litigation; gender-based asylum jurisprudence cases; and why some migration populations return to their native country for healthcare. At the conclusion of this chapter, the current and future trends in South African and American policy development vis-à-vis healthcare rights, asylum, enforcement, and litigation will be addressed.

THE PUSH AND PULL OF MIGRATION

Of the total world's population—some 6,853,328,460 as of 2010 census data—3.15% of the population, or about 215,738,321 are migrants, and 16.3 million are refugees and asylum seekers, some 8%, according to 2010 and earlier year statistics accumulated by peoplemovin via the World Bank Open Data, U.S. Census, and other immigration and refugee data compilation agencies (2013). As for our two population groups, Zimbabweans in South Africa and Mexicans in the U.S.A., both host countries (RSA and U.S.A.) see their chief immigration flows from these two countries (Zimbabwe and Mexico). Approximately 3.79%, or 1,862,889, of South Africa's population of 49,109,107 citizens are immigrants—with the vast bulk of them coming from Zimbabwe at 858,993—approximately 1.75% of the total population (compiled data as of 2010) (peoplemovin, 2013) (Figure 3.1).

In 2009, South Africa received over 222,000 new asylum requests (158,000 from Zimbabweans), which made RSA the No. 1 asylum destination of the world—over 25% of all global applications. The US was in second place, with less than 48,000 applications—one fifth the number of new individual asylum claims as SA (O'Connor 2010). The same report noted that 90% of Zimbabwean asylum claims globally were petitioned in South Africa in 2009, and as much as one-fourth of Zimbabwe's entire population has traveled to South Africa in recent years to flee ZANU-PF party violence and the dictatorial rule of President Robert Mugabe. According to UNHCR, South Africa's Department of Home Affairs, the government ministry assigned to oversee the

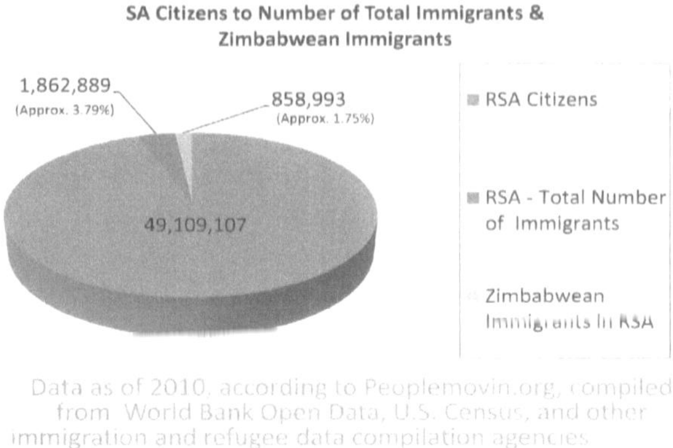

Figure 3.1 Immigration Profile: South Africa

asylum system, approved just 15.5% of the applications it processed in 2011, less than half the worldwide average recognition rate of 38% (IRIN 2013).

Conversely, approximately 13.79%, or 42,788,029, of the U.S.A.'s population of 310,232,863 citizens are immigrants—with the overwhelming majority arriving from México at 11,635,995—approximately 3.75% of the total population in U.S.A. (compiled data as of 2010) (peoplemovin 2013) (Figure 3.2). Statistics continue to show that few people seeking to flee the violence in Mexico are officially granted asylum in the United States. But while the number of Mexican asylum petitions approved by U.S. asylum officers and immigration judges in recent years has risen, it remains a mere minimal percentage of the multitude. In 2006, the U.S. received 2,793 applications and approved less than 2%, in 2007 again less than 2% were approved out of the 3,042 applications, while in 2008, 72 (or 2%) of the total 3,459 petitions received were approved, and finally in 2009, 62 (or 2.2%) of the total 2,816 petitions were granted full asylum status, according to data compiled from U.S. immigration courts by the Executive Office for Immigration Review under the U.S. Department of Justice (Ullo 2010). In 2012, about 15,284 Mexicans applied for U.S. sanctuary from persecution in Mexico, with a mere 418 successfully being granted asylum—with China topping all nationalities on political asylum permits in 2012 with 9,541 grantees out of 25,396 applicants (Freemantle 2013).

Clearly, the demand for immigration policies in every nation is driven by the "demand" for immigrants—whether as laborers, general demographic populist needs (specific age or sex group, such as young people or women), or other. One of the most intriguing comments I reviewed was by the International Organization for Migration's research study "*Assessing the Costs and Impacts of Migration Policy: An International Comparison*," edited by Solon

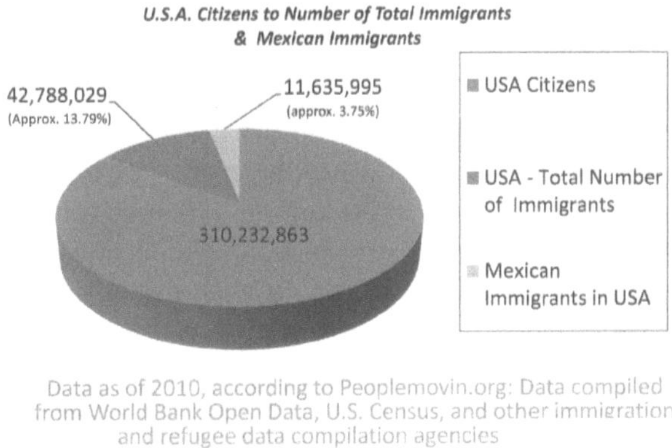

Figure 3.2 Immigration Profile: United States

Ardittis and Frank Laczko, which reviewed policies of several countries, stated the following broad-spectrum view of global immigration policies:

> Immigration policy, in particular, is seen as being about "who we are" as a nation. When there are no apparent problems with immigration generally, the policy is all but invisible. When there are problems—a major terrorist attack perpetrated by non-nationals or by naturalized individuals; race riots; a general sense of "otherness" based on, or giving rise to fears of the "difference" in cultures and religions, as seems to have been the case in the most developed world for about a decade now, immigration policy is seen as a crisis area and as something in which everyone wants a say because, indeed, it is seen as contributing to defining the nation. (2008, 15)

But with regard to illegal, unrecognized, or undocumented immigrants, the IOM report further points out that the "standard economic push factors" (such as higher expected income) drive much of the inflow. From the perspective of the receiving or "host" nation, undocumented migration is primarily determined by three critical factors: (1) proximity to source countries, (2) networks of existing legal and illegal immigrants, and (3) porous borders (IOM 2008). We certainly see all of these factors demonstrated in this piece of research targeting South Africa and the U.S.A. The "porous" or relatively unimpeded flow of undocumented migration across shared national borders, as well the huge pre-existing network of Mexican immigrants in the U.S. and Zimbabweans in South Africa—are all manifest and evident in this comparative analysis. Ardittis and Laczko's aforementioned book also attempted to "measure" national spending through evidence-based policymaking on immigration policy, focusing not only on a host nation's upfront administrative costs, but also the ongoing social, economic, and cultural integration costs of immigrant populations. According to the same book, there are three key dimensions in evaluating public spending on migration and asylum: evaluation of the policy's impact on immigrants and natives; a macroeconomic assessment of net social gains of the policies; and a cost-benefit assessment relative to the cost of each policy (based on a labor-market, family reunion, or asylum migration-driven system). Since data between various countries is many times non-comparable, the direct one-to-one evaluation of international policies is difficult. Since the "total impact" of immigration policy costs on a host (receiving) nation would entail analyzing immigration impacts on the labor market, product markets, welfare system, public revenues, capital stock, healthcare, education, and across numerous other public sectors, any truly comprehensive analysis would prove a burdensome task to accomplish, no matter the data comparability. In several noted studies, migration has been shown to only have a limited impact on a nation's healthcare system. One June 2009 study by Consortium for Refugees and Migrants in South Africa (CoRMSA) noted that the majority of cross-border immigrants are not seeking healthcare, but rather improved financial opportunities or an escape from political persecution. The consortium also reported that less than 50% of surveyed migrants reported a need for healthcare services in South Africa, with many reporting that they would return to their homeland for an illness that would preclude them from working. These reports dispute the oftentimes widespread public conjecture that foreign migrants suffer from poor health and drain a nation's already tightly strapped public health funds.

Refugees who seek permanent immigration status due to oppression, persecution, partisan-based violence, or maltreatment (such as torture, intimidation, feminine genital mutilation, imprisonment, etc.) in their native country are in yet another governmental and constitutional classification in the host country. In general terms, criteria for refugee determination are laid out in the 1951 United Nations Refugee Convention and also in the vast case law that has developed surrounding it. The definition of a refugee, according to the convention, is "a person who has a well-founded fear of being persecuted for reasons of race, religion, nationality, membership of a particular social group, or political opinion" (Dawes 2004, 252). Clearly, the use and the interpretation of broad-based terms like "well-founded fear," "particular," and "persecution" do little more than open up a veritable Pandora"s Box of opinions, miscommunication, and subjective interpretation for legal officers, nations, and refugee-seekers alike. Dawes goes on further to explain that these loosely interpreted terms can lead to wide-spread deception and fraud among refugee-seekers and legal officers. He noted that refugee seekers he saw at Human Rights Association, UNHCR, and International Committee of the Red Cross offices routinely attempted to "fix" and model their interview responses based on pre-determined and widely shared and published "successful" answers. Dawes noted that legal officers, as gatekeepers to the freedom of refugee resettlement, must readily dart the barbs of misused legalities and terminologies: "Manipulation and misinformation, is therefore, the background of their job" (2004, 252). Whether or not Dawes" statement on the integrity and scrupulousness of immigration officers holds true, both forced and voluntary migrants who are granted refugee status are exposed to an existence oftentimes mired in angst, insecurity, stress, and exploitation. As Edkins notes in "Sovereign Power, Zones of Indistinction, and the Camp," refugees in camps are turned into "invisible human beings, stateless, landless, and derelict," possessing nothing but bare life: "They were *homines sacri,*" people removed from the normal order and yet remaining in it (2000, 16). It is clear that migration bastions like South Africa and the U.S. are more likely to readily grant "humanitarian status" to Zimbabwean and Mexican undocumented migrants, rather than full-blown refugee status, so that the migrants hold little to no civil, legal, human, or healthcare rights, or any legal recourse to the denial of those rights.

POLICIES OF SOUTH AFRICA

According to "*Migrants' Right to Health in South Africa*" by George Mukundi Wachira of the Forced Migration Studies Programme at University of the Witwatersrand in Johannesburg, the right to life is the "most fundamental of all human rights, the supreme human right, and when a State does not recognize expressly the right to health, the duty of the State to ensure adequate access to essential care can be deducted by its obligation towards the right to life" (2009, 2). Furthermore, states Wachira, equality and non-discrimination provisions in all of the SADC nations' constitutions present a constitutional basis for migrants to claim their right to healthcare that is offered to citizens in their country of residence. Wachira also states that South Africa has 27 healthcare-related constitutional provisions, 24 HIV/AIDS specific laws and bills, 9 refugee-specific laws (including HIV prevention in prison), and 11 public health laws (including legislation of the National Health Act 61 of 2003).

In South Africa, the South African Constitution of 1996 guarantees everyone, citizens and migrants alike—regardless of legal status—"access to healthcare services" (Article 27–1) and forces the "state to take reasonable legislative and other measures within its available resources, to achieve the progressive realization of each of these rights" (Article 27–2) (South Africa Constitution 1996). The Constitution further stipulates that "no one is to be refused emergency medical treatment" and everyone is entitled to lifesaving care (Article 27–3) (1996). It should be noted that under the Refugees Act, legally recognized refugees are entitled to many other additional healthcare services, as well as non-citizens holding other permits in South Africa (CoRMSA 2009). The country's premiere national healthcare provider, the South African National Department of Health, set forth in 2008 that "refugees and asylum seekers—with or without a permit—should be assessed according to the current means test as applied to South African citizens when accessing healthcare" and that asylum seekers and refugees should not be charged "foreign category" fees (CoRMSA 2009). Furthermore, the nation's most basic constitutional rights to healthcare access have been solidified and substantiated through various national cases that have been brought to the South African Constitutional Court.

But the Consortium for Refugees and Migrants in South Africa (CoRMSA) report from June 18, 2009, notes that two key challenges outlined in their 2006, 2007, and 2008 reports continue to "remain problematic in 2009: (1) refugees and asylum seekers continue to have negative interactions with, experiences of, and treatment by, public healthcare providers (one-third reported challenges); and (2) ambiguity persists within the public system on refugees' and asylum seekers' rights to access healthcare in general and antiretroviral treatment (ART) in particular" (CoRMSA 2009). In the words of undocumented Zimbabwean 27-year-old "Jennifer," native South Africans make it clear publicly that refugees and/or immigrants from other countries are not readily welcomed and appreciated in their country: "They shout at us and some of them call us foreigners. They say we are taking their jobs. . . ." She said she is also very likely to be publicly taunted and hear the shouts of "*Makwerekwera!*" (a purportedly derogatory interlinguistic slang term for "foreigner," especially dark African immigrants) while she walks along the inner city streets of Johannesburg. (This South African term is adjusted and pronounced according to the native language of the speaker: A Zulu-speaker may pronounce it "*amakwerekwere,*" a Sotho-speaker may utter "*makwerekwere,*" and an English-speaker may drop the prefix entirely and verbalize only "*kwerekwere.*") Still, "Jennifer" said that she has no plans to return home and doesn't want to go back to Zimbabwe, and despite her current hardships and some on-the-street harassment by passersby in downtown Johannesburg, she likes her life as an undocumented Zimbabwean in South Africa. But these new residents are not always welcomed by their host country's residents. According to Aggad and Sidiropoulos, "These new arrivals have had a huge impact on South Africa's social landscape, including demand for jobs, housing, and other services; the results of the inflow include periodic outbreaks of tension that threaten to break out into open violence" (2008, 2). Undeniably, these tensions did lead to the outbreak of xenophobic violence in May 2008 that left dozens, reportedly about 60, people dead from attacks against immigrants and foreigners, and again in 2015.

As for international and regional human rights treatises relevant to migrants' right to healthcare in South Africa and the U.S.A., there are several worth noting due to their specific treatment of healthcare issues within each country's border. Since it would prove onerous to scrutinize each and every international, national, regional, and national protocol that can potentially affect asylum, emergency healthcare, and migration rights of female Mexican and Zimbabwean migrants in the U.S.A. and South Africa, this research will offer only an abridged inventory of the most significant healthcare, migration, gender-based political asylum, and human rights instruments adopted by South Africa and the U.S.A. The following excerpts are meant only to highlight the most pivotal, benchmark, and binding instruments affecting our two populations of undocumented Zimbabwean women in South Africa and undocumented Mexican women in the United States.

The following are selected (and not a comprehensive citation) of the ratified international instruments that speak to our two specific groups of forced migrant women, and their human and healthcare rights: Universal Declaration of Human Rights; the International Covenant on Civil and Political Rights (ICCPR); the International Convention on the Elimination of all Forms of Racial Discrimination (ICERD); the Convention Relating to the Status of Refugees; the International Convention on the Protection of the Rights of all Migrant Workers and Members of their Families (ICRMW); the International Covenant on Economic, Social and Cultural Rights (ICESCR); and the female-specific Convention on the Elimination of All Forms of Discrimination against Women (CEDAW).

To begin, no research on the topic of human rights can commence without at least a transitory nod to the Universal Declaration of Human Rights of 1948, proclaimed by the United nations General Assembly on December 10, 1948. This landmark and revolutionary document set out for the first time ever to globally protect human rights. Some 20 years later, in 1966, two treaties—one outlining civil and political rights (the International Covenant on Civil and Political Rights-ICCPR), and one addressing economic, social, and cultural rights (the International Covenant on Economic, Social and Cultural Rights—ICESCR)—were also adopted by the United Nations to form the supporting international keystones of human rights instruments. The 1966 International Covenant on Civil and Political Rights (ICCPR) was adopted by the UN General Assembly in December 1966 and adopted and opened for signature, ratification and accession by General Assembly resolution 2200A (XXI) on December 16, 1966, and entered into force in March 1976 (UNHR 2013). Over two decades later, this international covenant was ratified by the United States on June 8, 1992, and then signed by the Republic of South African government on October 3, 1994 (UNHR 2013). The ICCPR is based on the Universal Declaration on Human Rights, also known as the International Bill of Rights. In broad-based terms, the ICCPR commits its parties to respect the civil and political rights of individuals, rights which include the right to life, freedom of religion, assembly, association and speech, electoral rights and rights to due process and a fair trial. Even though the ICCPR does not contain specific provisions for safeguarding the right to health, it does indirectly link to healthcare rights via the right to life, non-discrimination and consent to medical and scientific experimentation. As of March 2010, the ICCPR had 72 signatories and 165 parties, according to the UN (2010). The ICCPR is monitored by the Human Rights Committee which oversees state reports, and rulings on complaints with regard to the alleged violations of the ICCPR submitted under the Optional Protocol to the Covenant (Wachira 2009).

After World War II (1914–1918), millions of refugees who had fled their homelands found themselves "stateless" and without travel documents or international status. So in 1951, the Convention Relating to the Status of Refugees was adopted on July 28 by the United Nations Conference of Plenipotentiaries on the Status of Refugees and Stateless Persons convened under General Assembly resolution of December 14, 1950, and was entered into force April 22, 1954 (UNHR 2013). The 1951 Refugee Convention is the fundamental legal document that set the parameters defining who should be classified a refugee, their rights, and the legal obligations of states. The government of South Africa signed the Convention Relating to the Status of Refugees on January 12, 1996. The subsequent 1967 Protocol amended and revised the 1951 Refugee Convention by eliminating some of the instrument's geographical and time-based limitations. This U.N. Protocol was voted into accession by the United States on November 1, 1968, however, with several notable reservations as follows:

> The United States of America construes Article 29 of the Convention as applying only to refugees who are resident in the United States and reserves the right to tax refugees who are not residents of the United States in accordance with its general rules relating to non-resident aliens. The United States of America accepts the obligation of paragraph 1 (b) of Article 24 of the Convention except insofar as that paragraph may conflict in certain instances with any provisions of title II (old age, survivors' and disability insurance) or title XVIII (hospital and medical insurance for the aged) of the Social Security Act. As to any such provision, the United States will accord to refugees lawfully staying in its territory treatment no less favorable than is accorded aliens generally in the same circumstances. (UNHR 2013)

The following year in 1969, the International Convention on the Elimination of all Forms of Racial Discrimination (ICERD) was entered into force on

January 4. ICERD specifically addresses the elimination of racial discrimination in public health and medical care access, attempting to eradicate racial disparities in health status as well as institutional racism within a healthcare system. This international convention was signed by the government of South Africa on October 3, 1994, and ratified on December 10, 1998, and then signed by the U.S. government on October 21, 1994, and ratified on September 28, 1996 (United Nations 2010). As of March 2010, ICERD had 85 signatories and 173 parties according to the U.N. (2010).

Later, in 1979, the female-specific Convention on the Elimination of All Forms of Discrimination against Women (CEDAW), which is often referred to as the "women's bill of rights," addressed maternal healthcare and other health-related issues. CEDAW was adopted by the UN General Assembly on December 19, 1979, coming into force as a treaty on December 3, 1981. CEDAW was signed by the government of South Africa on January 29, 1993, and ratified December 15, 1995 (United Nations 2010). Today it is one of the most broadly endorsed human rights treaties as it has been ratified or acceded to by 186 countries, constituting about 90% of the UN membership. It is here that we should note that as of August 2009, the United States is among a small minority of countries that have not yet ratified CEDAW, including Iran and Sudan. The United States has the appalling distinction of being the only country in the Western Hemisphere and the only industrialized democracy that has not ratified this treaty.

In 1990, the benchmark U.N. International Convention on the Protection of the Rights of all Migrant Workers and Members of their Families (UN document A/RES/45/158, also known as the "Migrant Workers Convention") was passed by the U.N. General Assembly in December of 1990, and formed new foundations, including the positioning of human rights (basic freedoms, due process, etc.) within the distinctive framework of documented and undocumented migrant rights. "As its salient feature, the Convention protects all migrant workers and members of their families, irrespective of their legal status. Nevertheless, the rights granted to documented and undocumented workers are not identical," according to Migrants Rights International (2013). At the time of this research's publication, neither South Africa nor the United States had signed or ratified this Convention.

When we move away from international and focus solely on (national) South African instruments, some (but not all) of the pivotal instruments that speak to migrants' and women's legal healthcare rights include: the SADC Protocol on Health; the OAU Convention Governing the Specific Aspects of Refugee Problems in Africa; the Refugees Act No. 130 of 1998; CoRMSA's "Gender Guidelines for Asylum Determination"; the African Charter on Human and Peoples Rights, and others. In 1981, the African (Banjul) Charter on Human and Peoples Rights is multinational human rights instrument whose purpose is to promote and protect human rights, including the right to life, in African nations. It was adopted on June 27, 1981, and entered into force on October 21, 1986. This Charter was signed by the government of South Africa in July 1996, and was ratified in July 1996. As of June 2009, 53 countries have ratified the charter (United Nations 2010).

The Republic of South Africa did not officially recognize refugees until 1993, after its shift to democracy, whereby it became a signatory to the United Nations and the Organization of African Unity Conventions on Refugees (OAUCR) (UNHR 2013). Some of South Africa's principal pieces of refugee and refugee healthcare protection legislation are the South African ACT 13–02 Immigration Act of 2002, Act No. 61 of 2003 7/18/2004, and National Health Act of 2004. The Refugees Act No. 130 of 1998, which sets forth the principles and standards relating to refugees, the provision for the reception of asylum seekers into South Africa, the regulation of applications and refugee status recognition, and the provision of rights and obligations for those immigration statuses. In general terms, these national instruments allow refugees who have been granted asylum (asylum applications should be adjudicated within 180 days, including any appeals) to apply for permanent RSA residence after five years of continuous residence, and only approved refugees are allowed to obtain for identity documents.

As for women's 2008 SADC Protocol on Gender and Development (August 17, 2008) looks into integration and mainstreaming of gender issues into the SADC Programme of Action and Community Building initiatives, attempting to provide for the empowerment of women, to eliminate discrimination, and realize gender equality via the creation and execution of gender-responsive legislation, procedures, and schemes. Articles 26 and 27 of the SADC Protocol on Gender and Development instruct States to tackle gender-specific HIV/AIDS healthcare needs, and open access to HIV/AIDS treatment for all who have been infected. The Republic of South Africa also accepted the "Gender Guidelines for Asylum Determination" penned by National Consortium on Refugee Affairs (CoRMSA) in 1999.

POLICIES OF THE U.S.A.

Concerning undocumented female migrants' legal healthcare rights within the U.S.A., the following international treatises have been ratified by the government of the United States of America: The 1996 International Covenant on Civil and Political Rights (ICCPR), and The International Convention on the Elimination of all Forms of Racial Discrimination (ICERD). The 1996 International Covenant on Civil and Political Rights (ICCPR) is ratified by both the U.S. and South African governments. This international covenant was signed by the government of the U.S.A. on October 5, 1977, and ratified on June 8, 1992. The International Convention on the Elimination of all Forms of Racial Discrimination (ICERD) is ratified by both the U.S. and South African governments. This international convention was signed by the U.S. government September 28, 1966, and ratified on October 21, 1994 (United Nations 2010).

In the United States, there have been several legal instruments that tackle immigration and claims for asylum. The United States' 1952 Immigration and Nationality Act (INA), Refugee Act of 1980, and Immigration Act of 1990 are the country's three pivotal national policy statements, addressing provisions of asylum, admissions, claims, and more. The Refugee Act of 1980 was enacted as an amendment to the Immigration and Nationality Act (INA) in order "to bring the United States into compliance with obligations" under the United Nations Protocol Relating to the Status of Refugees and the United Nations Convention (UNHR 2013). But before that, the 1952 Immigration and Nationality Act (INA) created the federal Immigration and Naturalization Service department, which was replaced by the Department of Homeland Security (DHS), and enforces immigration laws. The United States' Department of Homeland Security (DHS) was created in 2002, after the September 11, 2001, in which "four U.S. planes were hijacked by terrorists crashed into the World Trade Center, the Pentagon and a field in Pennsylvania killing nearly 3,000 people in a matter of hours," according to CNN (2013). With the passage of the Homeland Security Act by the U.S. Congress in November 2002, The DHS was created as a stand-alone, cabinet-level department and assimilated some 22 different federal departments and agencies into a singular unit, including U.S. Citizenship and Immigration Services (adjudications and benefits programs), U.S. Customs and Border Protection (inspection functions and the U.S. Border Patrol), and the U.S. Immigration and Customs Enforcement (immigration law enforcement: detention and removal, intelligence, and investigations) (DHS 2013). According to the DHS, only 11 days after the September 11, 2001, terrorist attacks, Pennsylvania Governor Tom Ridge was appointed as the first Director of the Office of Homeland Security in the White House, adopting and enforcing a national program to safeguard and respond to any future terrorist attacks. Within the U.S., there are several systems for the "checks and balances" to evaluate current pushes and international crises that drive migration policy. Some of the offices include the Government Accountability Office (GAO), the Department of Homeland Security (DHS) and various Congressional Commissions and evaluations (such as the U.S. Commission on Immigration Reform created in 1990), but some are U.S. government departments, such as Homeland Security, Health and Human Services (HHS), State, and Labor (IOM 2008). These four offices have conducted evaluations and studies that address migration and much of the evaluation in the United States is due to individual country-specific pieces of legislation, such as the Haitian Refugee Immigration Fairness Act of 1998.

Yet the escalating violence of the drug wars in Mexico continues to cause citizens to flee their country. Some continue to seek protection from the U.S. government as political refugees, even though the safeguard was initially intended to protect people who feared persecution from repressive governments. According to the U.S. Bureau of Citizenship and Immigration Services (USCIS), asylum seekers must demonstrate a "credible fear of persecution" in their country due to their race, ethnicity, religion, political views or social group (DHS 2013). If the U.S. started to grant political asylum in these cases, it would signify a drastic swing from its existing policy, as the majority of the asylum-seeking Mexicans are not fleeing their government, but violence from their own fellow citizens. Yet the formerly unyielding wall that has kept Mexicans from requesting political asylum has begun to show some minor cracks. In 2009, a former Mexican police officer named Guillermo Eduardo Ramirez-Peyro, who was paid $224,000 for information used to convict dozens of high-ranking Mexican narcotic smugglers, won his appeal at the U.S. Board of Immigration Appeals, as reported by *The Washington Times* (Seper 2009). His earlier denial for political asylum was overturned by the federal Eighth Circuit Court of Appeals, which found that asylum could be granted to him and others based on the Convention Against Torture. (Case 477 F.3d 637: Guillermo Eduardo Ramirez-peyro, Petitioner, v. Alberto Gonzales, Attorney General of the United States of America, Respondent. United States Court of Appeals, Eighth Circuit. Submitted: January 12, 2007, filed: February 23, 2007.) Seper's report noted that the court said that under the convention, "acquiescence by government officials that could lead to a petitioner's harm' was grounds to grant political asylum." Considered a noteworthy benchmark victory, the former Mexican police officer's bid for political asylum took over five years.

Recently, one significant step for immigration reform and a path to U.S. legalization was created on June 15, 2012, by President Barack Obama for undocumented Mexicans and other immigrants who were transported into the United States as children. Known as the Deferred Action for Childhood Arrivals (DACA) program, selected individuals who came to the United States as minors (under the age of 18) and meet seven guidelines can apply for this program for two years, and would then be eligible for work authorization if their status is renewed at that time. According to the United States department of Homeland Security and the U.S. Citizenship and Immigration Services (USCIS), "Deferred action is a discretionary determination to defer removal action of an individual as an act of prosecutorial discretion" (USCIS 2013, 1). The seven guidelines for undocumented immigrants (age 15 and up) are that the applicant is under the age of 31 (as of June 15, 2012); was brought into the U.S. before their 16th birthday; lived in the U.S. since June 15, 2012; were physically present in the U.S. at the time of your application and request; is in U.S. under expired or non-existent immigration status; enrolled in school or graduated from school; and without a felony conviction, three or more misdemeanor charges and not a threat to national or public safety (USCIS 2013). By March 2013, the USCIS reported that they had received 472,004 requests for the DACA program, and that 268,361 were approved, while 16,778 requests were rejected (temporarily) because they were judged to be incomplete, and 1,377 were denied, with the remaining applications under review—making for a very high 57% approval rating for the DACA applicants (Nevarez 2013). Yet the Deferred Action for Childhood Arrivals (DACA) program has ostensibly also produced an unpredicted dilemma: Since October, 2013, Texas' Border Patrol agents have made more than 170,000 arrests of illegal crossings, including 52,000 unaccompanied minors—an increase of 100% over 2012 (Usborne 2014). This record influx of migrants has led American leaders to brand it a far-reaching "humanitarian crisis" as it is stretching Texas, Arizona, and California immigration patrols, courts, and facilities far beyond their intended capacities.

For many Zimbabwean female migrants in South Africa, the words of Sefu (a refugee displaced by xenophobic violence who was turned away for care at Johannesburg General Hospital), echo the sentiment concerning the country's open access policies for healthcare: "Xenophobia is still here—only now it lives at the hospital" (Human Rights Watch 2009). In South Africa, Wachira notes that several legal cases have upheld migrants' rights to healthcare access and/or HIV treatment, including but is not limited to, the following cases: Mazibuko vs. Minister of Correctional Services and Others in 2007; EN and Others vs. Government of RSA and Others in 2007; Minister of Health and Others vs. Treatment Action Campaign and Others in 2002; and the Government of RSA and Others vs. Grootboom and Others in 2001. In some cases, reports have been recounted of undocumented Zimbabwean women being denied access to medication. As one example, in March 2012, Mai Tawanda, an HIV-positive Zimbabwean woman had to be "rescued" from Maitland Refugee Reception Centre in South Africa after she had been denied access to her antiretroviral drugs (Ndlovu 2012). According to Ndlovu's report, the NGO People against Suffering Oppression and Poverty (PASSOP) intervened after police ignored the woman's continual requests for ARV drugs. Of grave concern to these Zimbabwean deportees is not only the interruption of their medical treatment (which can have serious health implications), but access to similar medication and treatment in their homeland, as well as the dangerous potential development of a strain of anti-resistant HIV—each encompassing an incontrovertible prospect of death. Joao Biehl refers to these arenas (where neither legal/welfare nor medial institutions) directly intervene as a "zone of social abandonment" of ex-citizens (i.e. ex-humans) and these public "learned indifferences" to the population's plight leads to a (as Biehl unerringly dubs it) "socially authorized dying" (2005, 38).

In the U.S.A., undocumented migrants' right to healthcare access litigation is sporadic, ostensibly surrounding malpractice suits. For instance, on February 7, 2003, a 17-year-old undocumented Mexican teenager named Jesica Santillan (December 26, 1985—February 22, 2003) received a heart-lung transplant from Duke University in Durham, North Carolina. Two years prior, Jesica, two siblings, her mother, and her mother's boyfriend paid a smuggler (often called coyotes) some $5,000 to help them illegally enter the United States from Tamazula, Mexico, a town 275 miles west of Mexico City, so that Jesica could receive medical treatment for restrictive cardiomyopathy and (secondary) nonreactive pulmonary hypertension. Jesica was declared brain dead on February 20, as the Type A-blood type organs that had been transplanted did not match Jesica's type O-postive blood type, and the hospital's error in blood-typing was discovered shortly after the completion of her surgery. The Duke University Health System reached a sealed settlement (which also included an agreement that neither the hospital nor the family is allowed to comment on the case) and created a fund of $4 million to help other families of young Hispanic patients.

The American United Network for Organ Sharing (UNOS) is a non-profit organization that operates the Organ Procurement and Transplantation Network (OPTN) under contract with the U.S. Department of HHS, and was created by the Organ Transplant Act of 1984 by the United Network for Organ Sharing or UNOS (UNOS does not handle corneal donor tissue). A spokeswoman for the United Network for Organ Sharing was quoted by the Associated Press as saying they "cannot perform more than 5% of their transplants on noncitizens," and "federal law prohibits government reimbursement for organ-transplant-related services for undocumented aliens" (Irvine 2003). But when American medical facilities have tried to deny lifesaving organ transplants to illegal aliens, they have been met with both political, NGO, and media uproars. In 2012, a dying undocumented Mexican man living in California was denied a lifesaving kidney transplant due to his illegal status (Jennings 2012). This decision was later reversed by the hospital after his story was covered in the national media.

If we turn our focus toward gender-based asylum jurisprudence in the United States, a 1996 decision by the Board of Immigration Appeals (Case # A73 476 695) granted political asylum to Fauziya Kasinga, a young Togolese woman who feared genital mutilation in her home country. Prior to Kasinga's benchmark case, gender-based persecution as a basis for asylum in the United States was non-existent. Female genital mutilation (FGM) only became a tangible footing for asylum when American citizens found the practice appalling by social standards, and physically brutal and unnecessary by medical standards as to criminalize it domestically—thereby deeming it gender-based persecution whereby women are victimized by cultural practices that violate their human rights. The United States Board of Immigration Appeals (the nation's highest-authority immigration court) ruled that the FGM practice by the Tchamba-Kunsuntu tribe, constituted persecution, and that Kasinga had a well-founded fear of persecution due to her social group, and that her fear of persecution was country-wide, so therefore she qualified for political asylum (Neacsu 2013). Kasinga's case set the U.S. precedent and opened the doors for women to seek and acquire asylum on the basis of gender-related persecution due to rape, forced marriage, FGM, and honor crimes. In another high-profile and landmark gender-based persecution case, on April 27, 2011, the United States granted protection and stopped the forceful deportation of Tahirih (named as "A-T-") (cases: Matter of A-T-, 24 I&N December 296; Matter of A-T-, 24 I&N December 617; Matter of A-T-, 25 I&N December 4), according to the Tahirih Justice Center (2013). Tahirih had already undergone the FGM procedure in her native country of Mali, but feared further persecution and a forced marriage from her social group. It should be noted that gender-based primary violence, such as spousal abuse or FGM, is generally only considered grounds for asylum when it is so severe and unconscionable that it would constitute persecution. It should also be noted that the woman's government is found to be either unwilling or unable to protect her from her persecutor(s), and the persecution is inflicted due to the five characteristics protected by the United States' law of asylum: political opinion, race, nationality, religion, or membership in a particular social group. Therefore, many applicants' cases are initially rejected by the primary trial (district, circuit or superior or "lower") courts and then appealed until they reach the appellate ("higher") courts, a protracted and expensive process of litigation that can take numerous years.

POLICY ENFORCEMENT AND LITIGATION

Even individual states in America are making big independent moves in immigration and large-scale social reform legislation. In April 2010, the U.S. Arizona State Senate voted to approve the final version of a bill that would impose some of the toughest immigration laws in the country, which would give police broad new powers to arrest and charge people suspected of being in the country illegally, according to Fox News (2010). Some of the never-before-seen in the U.S. provisions and parameters include: a new state misdemeanor crime for failing to carry alien registration documents; the ability of officers to arrest immigrants unable to show documents proving their legal residence; the allowance of people to sue if they feel a government agency has adopted a policy that hinders immigration enforcement; the prohibition of people from blocking traffic when they seek or offer day labor services on street corners; and charges for people to knowingly transport illegal immigrants (Fox News 2010).

In April 2012, a Republican Texas State Representative from San Antonio, Lyle Larson, sent a letter to Mexican President Felipe Calderon asking for Mexico to reimburse Texas for services used by illegal Mexican migrants. According to the *Daily Caller* newspaper, Larson invited Mexico to pay Texas back the annual $6 billion to $8 billion that the state of Texas spends on healthcare, education and other public services for the estimated 1.6 million undocumented Mexican immigrants in the state, Larson explained. "If Mexico is unable to provide monetary compensation, we should be open to discussing other forms of payment . . . by allowing U.S. companies to develop mineral rich areas of northern Mexico and collect these resources as an in-kind payment," thus providing "high-paying jobs for Mexican citizens, while allowing Mexico to pay Texas back for the services we are rendering to citizens of your country," stated Larson (May 2012, 1). Even in natural disasters, undocumented immigrants in the U.S. face a thorny new future. For instance, in the case of an evacuation from a hurricane, in Texas' Rio Grande Valley, all residents will be checked for a citizenship by U.S. Customs and Border Patrol as they attempt to flee a natural disaster (Brezosky 2008). According to the report, U.S. Customs and Border Protection has confirmed it will check the citizenship both of people boarding buses to leave the area and at inland traffic checkpoints, and anyone determined to be in the country illegally or without proper citizenship status will be taken to detention centers away from the hurricane's path and processed for deportation. Every year, the U.S. Customs and Border Protection, hospitals, state governments, and the U.S. Department of the Interior face litanies of lawsuits filed by (or on behalf of) undocumented Mexican aliens in the U.S.A. In May 2012, families of 11 Mexican immigrants who died of dehydration illegally crossing the Arizona-Mexican sued two U.S. federal agencies for $41 million dollars—claiming that U.S. Fish and Wildlife Service personnel failed to provide "humane" water stations for the people (Miller 2012). The same report also noted that each immigrant had paid $1,400 for the illegal crossing through a remote 860,000-acre wildlife refuge, and their deaths were added to the number of 1,000+ immigrants annually who die attempting to cross into the U.S. illegally. In a curious and rather extraordinary twist of "reverse migration," it is the Americans who are in fact crossing the U.S.-Mexican border to seek out inexpensive drugs and take advantage of the low-cost medical tourism development in Mexico. Again, is the Americans (who seemingly can no longer to afford to pay for "*the greatest healthcare system in the world*") who are traveling abroad to Mexico, Thailand, Singapore, and India for elective surgery and care. These Americans, who in many reports and studies conceded to tiring of the distressing American medical industry's (sardonically dubbed) "wallet biopsy," were willing to forgo the high-tech (i.e. high cost) scientific innovations in the United States and take their chances with more affordable (yet perhaps less closely regulated or reputable) care outside of the United States. Mexican doctors and dentists can operate at much lower costs in that they do not need to purchase medical malpractice (improper, unskilled, or negligent treatment of a patient by a physician, dentist, nurse, pharmacist, or other healthcare provider) insurance. According to Reuters news service, an average of 10 cents from every dollar spent on American healthcare goes directly into the coffers of malpractice insurance costs—just in case the patient ever tries to sue them (Furchtgott-Roth 2009). The cost of malpractice insurance in the United States varies by two primary factors: the doctor's specialty (area or practice) and the state in which the doctor is licensed and offers medical care. Malpractice insurance premiums in the U.S. are the highest among neurosurgical and obstetrical specialties due to the prevalence of neurological-based chronic pain, paralysis, and long-term disabilities—and obstetrical-based prenatal and perinatal factors that can lead to maternal death, fetal death (stillborn), cerebral palsy (incurable brain and nervous system function disorders that can be caused by lack of oxygen during the birth process that affects movement, learning, hearing, seeing, and thinking), and other birth injuries and defects that can involve lifelong care and expensive restorative treatment. Insurance premiums in malpractice can range from $4,000 for family practitioners in a low-cost state to $200,000 and more in a high-cost state for an OB/GYN. American malpractice litigation costs hit over $30 billion a year in 2009, with litigation taking a minimum of three years, and since 1975 direct costs of litigation avoidance have grown at more than 10% annually (Furchtgott-Roth 2009).

In Tena-Tamayo's article, "Malpractice in Mexico," the author, who is the National Commissioner for Medical Arbitration in Mexico, describes how doctors are forced to buy expensive malpractice insurance, which seriously affects their medical practice by distorting it into what the author dubs as "defensive medicine." Tena-Tamayo explains how the ever-constant apprehension of malpractice litigation keeps American doctors mired in "defensive medicine"—a costly and preventable contest whereby doctors and patients suffer, and attorney and insurance corporations' profit:

> The growing number of lawsuits against doctors seems to be related to poor personal communication, unrealistic expectations of performance, the high costs of medical attention, and better informed and more critical patients. A lucrative industry has developed around this phenomenon. In response, doctors buy

> expensive insurance, which seriously affects their medical practice, summarized in the concept of "defensive medicine." The practice of defensive medicine includes ordering excessive diagnostic procedures and consultations to minimize the risks of being sued. Consequently, the cost of medical care increases, promoting resentment in patients, which in turn favors lawsuits, creating a vicious circle. Fear of being sued drives some doctors to additional detrimental actions, such as abandoning risky specialties; refusing to treat seriously ill patients; and using clinical records and informed consent forms as means of legal protection, rather than as medical tools. Differentiation between complications (an unintentional or adverse reaction that aggravates the original disease) and negligence (failure to exercise a reasonable degree of care) is not always simple and may be interpreted differently by the doctor and the patient or their legal adviser. (Tena-Tamayo 2005, 1)

Tena-Tamayo's so-called "vicious circle" of medical malpractice is not followed in his native country of Mexico, a country that chooses mediation and arbitration, not litigation. The commissioner claims that Mexico's methods accelerate the resolution of conflicts, are less costly, discourage "trivial lawsuits," allow arbiters with some medical knowledge (rather than lawyers), and in the end ". . . although the total amount awarded is usually less than that awarded by a judicial court, lawyer contingency fees and court costs are avoided" (2005, 1). For instance, Mexican dentists regularly charge one-fifth to one-fourth of U.S. dental care charges, and 45% of the American population has no dental insurance (Roig-Franzia 2007). American-based retirement communities are organizing bus tours for Mexican dental work, inexpensive drugs, and cheap healthcare.

Our interviews reflected that many of the undocumented Mexican women questioned for this research considered American healthcare to possess a callous, profit-driven "big business" approach: "[American] Doctors make business with diseases and sickness. And they don"t give you the necessary treatment so you'll come back and pay more," explained a 27-year-old female. A 19-year-old undocumented woman diagnosed with thyroid cancer stated, "It is difficult to get treatment in this country because it is expensive. . . . They were nice and good to me. I still talk with a nurse from the hospital [in Texas]. But my treatment was too expensive and I had to travel back to Mexico to continue with my [cancer] treatment." And yet another woman explained, "They [the hospital] said I owe less than $5,000. I felt like I was lost. . . . I couldn't think what I would do to pay the money," stated a 42-year-old undocumented Mexican woman who was treated in an emergency room for complications from Hepatitis B at a Houston-area hospital.

In conclusion, several reports have shown that Zimbabwean patients continue to be denied care, charged exorbitant and usury fees, subjected to long delays, extortion, and/or improper healthcare treatment, or prematurely discharged—making healthcare unrealizable for many migrants. These policies not only reflect a violation of medical ethics, but a violation of the South African Constitution. The government of South Africa must do more to confirm that hospital and clinic healthcare staff is cognizant and mindful about the rights of refugees, asylum-seekers, and migrants to access the RSA public health system, regardless of their legal status. Additionally, all ancillary and/or specialized care clinics and providers should allow for the free access and treatment of Zimbabweans who cannot afford it.

In the reconsideration of the curious new waves of cross-migration of some Americans into Mexico to seek low-cost healthcare—coupled with the return of some ill Mexicans themselves—collectively beg the question: If the United States claims to have (one of) the best healthcare systems in the world, the flow of cross-border healthcare-seeking behavior would be solely unidirectional, with both populations swarming into the United States . . . but they aren't. Hence the fiscal pendulum of access and provision of American "defensive healthcare" has begun to swing wildly out of balance, with no equilibrium or stability between feasible cost and sustainable care. Yet the access of migrants to high-cost, high-tech emergency healthcare continues to be kept in check, to some degree, in part to the hyper-litigious American environ and easy access to lawyers and advocate groups who will sue on behalf of the plaintiff (oftentimes without any upfront cost) for malpractice (criminal medical malpractice, or compensatory or punitive damages, etc.), revocation of licensure, and civil and/or criminal litigation.

At its quintessence, migration can either provide a constructive economic and social impact through a vibrant labor force, and rich cultural communities, or it can have negative effects such as human trafficking, labor exploitation and welfare and healthcare fraud. Most typically, migration produces both good and bad corollaries. Immigration policies in the United States and South Africa should be considered as critical and paramount to its citizenry as federally mandated education, healthcare, and defense stratagems. What seems sorely lacking is the establishment of adequate and data-comparable evaluation systems that would execute and facilitate all stages of policy formation and implementation. However, this means that countries must first question whether their policies are going to focus foremost on serving and defending their own national interests—or will they incorporate region-conscientious "Good Samaritan" humanitarian and development policies? Then the countries must strive to publicly (nationally) and globally articulate those fundamental goals. What is certain is that immigration and asylum policies cannot be evaluated solely via economic terms when there are numerous human rights, international security, public health, education, and national identity issues that must be weighed and kept in balance. Moreover, migration policies should stop ascertaining their effectiveness based solely on a high-income country's own national interest, but rather approach migration and asylum policy as intertwined regional and global policies that affect employment, education, foreign affairs, development, and healthcare access. There remains a great potential for courts and international conventions to improve fair access within each country's system and to decrease inequalities through the interpretation of existing legislation and in both of these jurisdictions. Each nation's willingness to do so hinges on the country's ongoing commitment and conviction in their role concerning the public's access to emergency healthcare. The voices and experiences of these undocumented women should be told, and we will listen to some of them now.

Chapter 4

Voices of the Women

Due to a lack of significant and current gender-based (or gender-disaggregated) refugee and forced migrant research that explores dual countries' undocumented healthcare policies, a small sampling of one-on-one interviews was undertaken for this piece of research itself. The rationale behind the creation of the interviews is that gender-specific dialogues must be collected in order to identify and establish particular gender-based differences in the treatment, behaviors, opportunities, and vulnerabilities of undocumented and forced migrant females that seek out emergency health care. The intention of these interviews was not to provide conclusive endorsements of particular migration policies, but rather to serve as an illustration of how inequitable power relations can impact undocumented women's health care and access. This chapter's information hopes to lay the groundwork for future research as well as assist emergency healthcare planners and providers to adequately plan for women in future forced migration scenarios and disasters.

The initial section of this chapter will address the six dimensions of each woman's emergency healthcare experience in her "Gender, Social Justice, and Healthcare Interview" (Appendix A—in English, Shona and Spanish languages). The queries are targeted to ascertain each woman's role as a decision-maker in seeking emergency medical care; barriers to obtaining care; assessment of accessibility, availability, quality, equity, and credibility of care; usage of the services; assessment of provider response; and gender-equitable treatment throughout the process. This will be followed by firsthand accounts of the interviews in a written monologue fashion, including both direct and indirect quotes from the women obtained during their interviews. Next we will look at some of the limitations of the interviews and any significant lessons we learned from creating and executing the various interview sessions. Lastly, we will focus on the chasm between theoretical healthcare rights and practical effects of those rights. As witnessed through these interviews, the reality of many forced migrants' experiences in claiming their accorded host country's healthcare rights was more theoretical than practical in its dispensation.

The sampling and methodologies chosen for this work include theoretical research, practical fieldwork experience, interviews with healthcare providers, and brief (one-day) healthcare interviews among a randomly solicited (previously unacquainted) group of female Mexican and Zimbabwean refugees who had sought and utilized emergency healthcare services as unrecognized refugees. These 24 interviews will hopefully provide useful insight into the women's experiences, as well as gender-based information essential for scholarly study and mainstream public media attention. The 24 interviews involved one-on-one anonymous "snowball sampling" interviews with female refugees who have previously accessed or attempted to access emergency healthcare services in the U.S.A. (Mexican undocumented migrants in Houston, Texas) and South Africa (Zimbabwean forced migrants in Johannesburg).

At this time, it would behoove this research to address any issues concerning the number of interviews in this research. To address the critical issue of sample size, a much more in-depth explanation of the research's methodological pluralism, ethics, seven interview criteria, and the interview selection processes are to be clarified, delineated, and expanded upon at this time. First, it is imperative to note that none of the volunteer interview subjects were ever recruited, spoken to, and/or communicated with inside or outside or anywhere near or on the premises of any healthcare facility or emergency care clinic in either Houston or Johannesburg. At no time were any of the women interviewed my former patients, acquaintances, or former patients of fellow healthcare providers, etc. None of the women who volunteered for the interviews were previously known or familiar to me, either privately (via friends, acquaintances, etc.) or publicly (through NGO services, medical care or academic institutions, etc.). At no time was the privileged information or communication between myself as a healthcare practitioner and a patient utilized whatsoever, ensuring total client confidentiality, health information privacy and protection, and provider-patient privilege and privacy. At no time were the interviewees or interviewee's family/friends solicited or given any fiscal reimbursement, aid, or beneficiary considerations whatsoever, either from me or anyone who was/is affiliated with an NGO I worked with at any time. Second, the explanations behind the sample size are easily explained as the sample was publicly solicited, and each interviewee had to meet over seven mandatory and strictly enforced criterions, as listed below. Please note that each and every of the following seven criteria were required to be present in order to utilize a singular subject. (1) Volunteer subject must be female. (2) Volunteer subject must be either (a) a Mexican or (b) a Zimbabwean national and had to have resided in the country of Mexico or Zimbabwe as an adult (over 18 years old)—if subject only had experience as a (minor under 18 years of age) as a resident, then interviewee was not chosen. (3) Volunteer subject must have sought out emergency care only in host country of South Africa or U.S.A.—excluding any ongoing care, non-emergency, or long-term treatment for chronic condition-care such as HIV/AIDS, or TB, or other long-term health/disease issue(s). The interviewee must have not only sought out care, but presented herself as a patient in need of emergency assistance at an emergency room/facility in either the city of Johannesburg or Houston. (4) Volunteer subject must be over 18 years (currently at the time of interview) *and* at the time of emergency care—no minors or care experience(s) as a minor would be accepted. (5) Volunteer subject must not be currently (or have been in the past) a patient or present/past recipient of any aid, fiscal reimbursement, or medical care of an NGO provider or myself at any time whatsoever. (6) Volunteer subject must currently be undocumented (in host country) at time of interview *and* at the time of the emergency care. (7) After meeting all of the above mandatory criteria, the volunteer subject had to be found compliant, disposed of (time-wise), be found mentally fit to understand/reply to queries, and amenable to the interview. Third, it is again significant to unequivocally state that none of the interviewed or women for/in this research were at any time my patients or received any aid, fiscal compensation, or direct or indirect recompense from me or anyone affiliated with our NGO or NGO's work. None of the subjects who are subjects in this research were at any time the interviewed subjects or family members/friends of the interviewed subjects.

At its core, the "Gender, Social Justice, and Healthcare Interview" (see Appendix A for English, Shona, and Spanish language translations) queries are targeted to ascertain the six following dimensions of women's experiences in: (1) a woman's active or passive role as a decision-maker in seeking and obtaining emergency medical care for herself; (2) assessment of realized, potential, and/or perceived physical, financial, physiological, informational, mental, and social barriers to obtaining and receiving EMS care as a refugee or undocumented immigrant; (3) their assessment of accessibility, availability, quality, equity (or any discrimination or discriminatory practices, such as excessive fees, racism, etc.), and credibility of EMS care and treatment; (4) their usage of the healthcare services, delineated between illnesses (diseases) and injuries (trauma-related), as well as major categories of medical practices (obstetrics, oncology, surgery, pharmaceutical, respiratory, etc.); (5) their assessment of EMS and healthcare provider response (as effective or non-effective) and treatment (respect, courtesy, racism, etc.); and

(6) women's assessment of gender-equitable and fair treatment in triage and screening processes, EMS, healthcare aid distribution, counseling, and more.

The interviews themselves were conducted on a personal one-to-one basis, with only women who have personally received or attempted to receive emergency healthcare services participating in the three-page, 23-question interview, which was written in a very simplified text and a simple (elementary/primary school) reading level of English and translated into Shona and Spanish. The translated interviews proved very necessary to have for the Spanish translators in the U.S.A., but the vast majority of the Zimbabwean women exhibited a solid working knowledge of English, but a translator was available at all times in case there was a need for explanation or further translation.

The Mexican women's interviews were conducted in Houston, Texas, at a southwest homeless shelter and a Hispanic-led church facility in southeast Houston. For instance, at the church, a call for potential interviewees was advertised via a spoken appeal for volunteers prior to one Sunday's church service. In contrast to their Zimbabwean counterparts, the Mexican women exhibited a very insufficient understanding of the English language and the vast majority of the interviews, with the exception of only two, were all conducted in Spanish with (later) written translations. The Mexican women were residing in Houston, known for its copious proportions of Hispanic populations—thus the explainable lack of need for English language skills among the women. Houston is the fourth largest city in America, with 2.1 million people within an area of 579 square miles (1,500 sq. km). There are more than 100 hospitals in the Houston area, which is widely renowned for its Texas Medical Center that boasts M.D. Anderson, the U.S.A.'s top cancer center, and Memorial Herman Hospital's Life Flight, one of the nation's best medical air ambulance services. The city also lists some 266 private air and road ambulance services, not including citywide firefighter/paramedic units on emergency "9-1-1" call standby.

The Zimbabwean women's interviews were conducted in Johannesburg, South Africa, via advertised calls for participation through the Central Methodist Church, the Jesuit Refugee Centre, South African Volunteers in Mission (SAMVIM), and Restoration of Human Rights (ROHR) Zimbabwe. Through my friends and acquaintances, several sessions were made every year to interview several women that had sought out emergency health care in South Africa. All of the undocumented women were residing in Johannesburg at the time of their interviews. The city of Johannesburg has a population of approximately 2.4 million stretching over 424.7 square miles (1,100 sq. km). Johannesburg comprises approximately 40 public and private hospitals, including the Chris Hani Baragwanath Hospital in Soweto, which is equipped with 4,000 beds and is one of the largest hospitals of the world.

IN THEIR OWN WORDS

This research compiled a small interview sampling of 10 undocumented female Mexicans living in Houston, Texas, and 14 undocumented Zimbabwean women living in Johannesburg, South Africa. Both Houston and Johannesburg are considered large, sprawling urban cities that attract inordinately large numbers of undocumented foreign residents and refugees. When contrasted, the group of interviewed Zimbabwean women had sought out emergency care 16 times more than their interviewed Mexican female counterparts, with the interviewed Zimbabwean women totaling an average of 4.8 visits, while the interviewed Mexican women only averaged 2.3 visits. While the average age of the interviewed undocumented woman was comparable at 31 years (31.1) for Zimbabwean women and 33 years (33.9) for the Mexican women, their lengths of stay differed drastically, with Zimbabwean women at a mere 10.7 months, as compared to the interviewed Mexican women's stay of 6.8 years (or 81.6 months). (See 'Undocumented Zimbabwean and Mexican Women—Months in Host Country,' Figure 4.1.)

Nonetheless, the considerable disparity in these numbers may have a rather uncomplicated answer, conceivably relatively easily attributed to the locations where the random interviews took place. For the Zimbabwean women, interviews were solicited through ROHR Zimbabwe, the Jesuit Refugee Center, and the Central Methodist Church—all three providing sanctuary and aid as first initial "starting points" for recent Zimbabwean refugees. For the Mexican women, interviews were solicited through Crossroads at Park Place Ministry, and a Houston-based urban Catholic church that preferred to remain anonymous. The Houston locations—including a large urban aid outreach

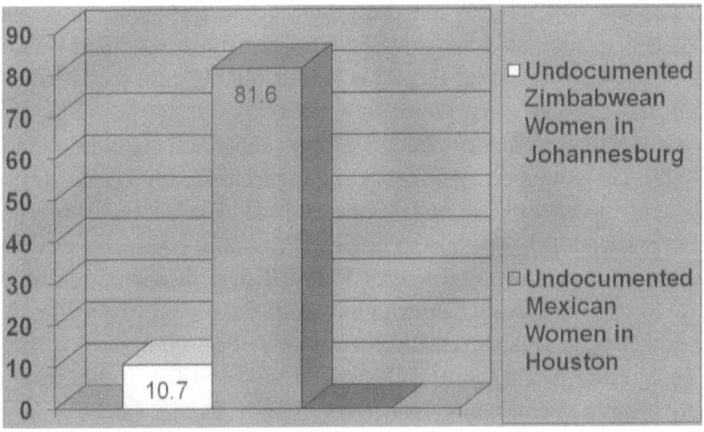

Figure 4.1 Surveyed Undocumented Zimbabwean and Mexican Women—Months in Host Country

could be deemed as service, NGO, and religious organizations that cater to somewhat (more) established and stable familial communities.

Through these interviews I uncovered three women's experiences that proved to be a 'common thread'—shared among many of the undocumented Mexican women who found themselves unable to afford America's high-cost health care and incapable of receiving federal, state, or local healthcare aid as undocumented residents. They are the voices of Mary, Norma, and Zoila. Maria, a 38-year-old mother of three, like many of the other interviewed Mexican women, sought out county- or state-run funded care at Strawberry Health Center (Pasadena, Texas) and other larger public hospitals like Lyndon Baines Johnson (LBJ) General Hospital, University of Texas-Medical Branch (UTMB) (Galveston, Texas), or Ben Taub (the largest public Level I trauma center in Houston). Mary said she suffered with severe gynecological issues for over a year before a physician at Memorial Hermann finally approved her to receive the necessary surgical intervention she needed. Maria also reported to have lost confidence in American hospitals and physicians and cited depression, money worries, and a fear of deportation due to her undocumented immigration status as key stressors: "You need a Gold Card [Harris County Texas healthcare aid program] or legal documents for everything here!"

Norma, like Maria, became ill and sought out emergency care first at the Strawberry Health Center, and then she was taken to LBJ Hospital in Houston for long-term care. She was diagnosed with inflammation of the liver and put in quarantine after she was diagnosed with Hepatitis. Several other people she was in contact with also tested positive for the contagious viral infection and they were also immediately quarantined. When I asked Norma if she had developed Hepatitis A, B, or C, she was unsure which form she had contracted. But she remembered her exact liver count and some other numbers from her test results, so I would surmise from those specified diagnostics that she had contracted either Hepatitis B (most likely case scenario from her short hospital stay) or even Hepatitis C (less likely, yet possible—a strain with much longer term health effects). Norma explained that while she was in the hospital, she struggled with fiscal and communication issues, explaining that: "I cannot speak English and no one told me what happened to me. They didn't bring someone to explain to me, I didn't know what they were saying. I felt like lost . . . . They said it was $5,000 I owe. I couldn't think what I would do to pay the money," Norma reported.

Like both Norma and Mary, Zoila could also ill afford high-cost American health care. Zoila is a 43-year-old married mother of four children, living in suburban area surrounding Houston. After living in the U.S. for seven years, Zoila has only recently attempted to access emergency health care in America. Zoila has a long history of gynecological issues, and she recently sought care due to spasms and severe gynecological symptoms. Since she has no healthcare insurance, she called upon a local clinic branch of UTMB, which she thought would help her. The woman working UTMB's patient intake said she needed a minimum of $25,000 before they would take her as a patient: "I feel free to ask for help. The doctor is a doctor, he is not the government . . . I try to live like the people here. I love the United States and they give you a lot of things but they don't let me be free and get social security [federal benefits]. I told my sister I think we have to go back to Mexico and she started to cry." But Zoila also reported that racism is the reason she has fear, and worries for her family's safety in the United States. She reported that 5 or 6 African-American men attacked her Hispanic son, kicking and beating him so severely that he needed to seek emergency medical care for his injuries.

Similar to Zoila, Leslie reported that she has been a victim of racism, and fears deportation and the 'money-hungry' American healthcare system. Leslie is a 27-year-old mother of one who has sought out emergency care on several occasions for recurrent abdominal pain, diarrhea, migraines, and coughing. Leslie said that even though the hospital staff was helpful, she had to find funds, about $175 U.S. Dollars, in order to purchase expensive medicines prescribed by the doctors. "American doctors make businesses with diseases and sicknesses. They don't give you the necessary help and medicines so you'll come back and pay more again . . . I feel sad and lonely," she reported.

Four of the interviewed undocumented Mexican women specifically reported domestic abuse by their spouse or their ex-spouse (also children's fathers). Maria, Elena, and Elizabeth are three examples of the women who claim to live in fear due to physical abuse—one even resulting in corporal trauma so severe that she needed to seek out emergency care in the United States. Maria, a 45-year-old woman with two minor (under 18 years old) children, claims that she "worries for her safety" as her husband beats her. Maria is one of the women who claimed depression as a reason she has sought out medical care in Houston, where she lives with five other people in her home. Maria went to the UTMB once in Galveston, Texas, to seek emergency care for, "being hurt by another person." The second time she sought out emergency care was illness and discomfort due to a high-risk pregnancy. During her obstetrical care, Maria said she was found to have uterine cancer and she has continued to receive oncological treatment under Medicaid. Maria said she is now healthy and the hospital staff was "very nice" to her during the treatment.

Like Maria, 36-year-old Elena claims she is a victim of domestic violence from her "aggressive" husband. But unlike Maria, Elena, who is a mother of four, said her emergency care in Houston was a dreadful experience. Less than two months pregnant, Elena claims she sought emergency care for vaginal bleeding at LBJ General Hospital in Houston. Elena claims she waited over 8 hours at the overcrowded LBJ emergency room, only to lose her baby due to obstetrical complications. Elena explained: "As a patient, you have to wait unless you are dying! . . . The doctors took a long time for [sic] attending to me and I lost the baby." She said she is depressed and has lost confidence in the American healthcare system and its providers. Elena blames her lack of timely obstetrical care in the emergency room on the loss of her baby, though she could not specifically explain nor relate the exact medical causes of the stillbirth.

Comparable to both Maria and Elena, is 31-year-old Elizabeth, a mother of two, who said that the father of one of her son's physically menaces, threatens, and frightens her. Elizabeth said her baby's father (they are unmarried) is brutal and cruel to her, and she lives in persistent fear of domestic violence from him. Moreover, Elizabeth had a very negative healthcare experience at a local Houston hospital (UTMB) in Galveston, Texas: "I was mistreated during the delivery and they did not apply anesthesia. All of the hospital rooms were occupied, so I had to deliver in a provisional room." Elizabeth also reported that she was depressed and lonely, and despite all of her adverse encounters in the United States—incessantly fears deportation back to Mexico.

It is consequential to note that all four of the Mexican women who reported domestic abuse also had cited depression as the one (or the only) illness that they sought medical attention for in the U.S.A. This is a significant finding in that domestic abuse can lead to emotional turmoil, melancholy, social isolation, and depression. (It should also be observed that 3 out of these 4 Mexican women also noted that they [additionally] bore financial troubles and immigration/deportation anxieties.) According to a 2010 report on "Depression Caused by Domestic Abuse" finding: "Adult women who have been abused in a relationship in the past five years have rates of depression 2 ½ times greater than women who have never been abused . . . They are also more likely to be socially isolated," said Amy Bonomi, associate professor at The Ohio State University. The same report noted that the mental health consequences of domestic violence include depression, as well as anxiety disorders, suicide, eating disorders, and substance abuse (Bonomi 2010). These findings would conspicuously point to plausible explanations to elucidate why depression was reported by these specified women.

The vast majority of the interviewed Zimbabwean women had survived various episodes of armed robbery, unarmed theft, assault (physical and/or sexual), and police (or border guard or some "authority figure") corruption, harassment, theft, or embezzlement. Out of the 14 interviewed Zimbabwean women, 5 feared "for their safety" and 6 had been the victim of police (or "authority") corruption, theft, harassment, or assault. Maria, a 20-year-old single unmarried mother of one child, lives at Central Methodist Mission Church and doesn't feel safe at the church or in South Africa. She has been a victim of theft, assault, and violence. After six months in South Africa, she has accessed emergency medical care about five times, primarily due to a pregnancy and her new baby's illness. At the interview, Maria had just given birth to a baby girl four months ago. She had initially sought emergency medical care from Hillbrow Hospital due to severe back pain during her pregnancy. The first two times she went to Hillbow, she was turned away without any triage or patient assessment. On the third encounter, she was in active labor and called an ambulance, but the ambulance service refused to come to the church. She then took a taxi cab to Hillbrow, and had the baby at the hospital, spending the day after the birth in the hospital. After the baby's birth, Maria took the child to Coronation Hospital, taking a taxi, and her child received medical care for free. On the second visit to Coronation with a sick baby, the child was treated initially for pneumonia and then for tuberculosis. The baby stayed in the hospital for a full week, and Maria stayed with the infant in the hospital. At the time of the interview, Maria and the baby had just been released from the hospital the previous day. "I don't feel safe here," Maria said. There's a lot of fighting and Maria has had things stolen from both her and her child.

Twenty-three-year-old Pretty, like Maria, has been also been assaulted. Pretty is a married mother of one child, living at the Central Methodist Mission Church. After four months in South Africa, she has accessed emergency medical care three times, due to her baby's illness, her own illness, and an incidence of assault. Two months ago, in an attempted theft, another resident beat Pretty to the extent that she not only sought emergency medical care, but also reported the assault to the Johannesburg police. The police gave her paperwork which allowed her to seek medical treatment. Pretty did seek help at Hillbrow Hospital, but was turned away: "'Go back to Zimbabwe' they said to me." When she and her baby were ill, both Joubert Park Municipal Clinic and Hillbrow Hospital turned them away, refusing to triage (check vital signs or any patient intake record) or care for either. But when she approached the local MSF Clinic, she and her child were treated with kindness and given free medication. She explained that she is now scared of the government and no longer trusts hospitals in South Africa. She had 12 years of education in her native country of Zimbabwe, but has not found a job or a place, other than the church, to stay in South Africa: "At first it was very hard to sleep here . . . But I feel sad about being here."

Like Pretty, the words Constance remembers the Hillbrow Hospital admissions clerk repeatedly shouting at her were: "You have no papers! We don't assist people from Methodist!"—An obvious reference to Central Methodist Church, where hundreds of Zimbabweans find refuge in downtown

Johannesburg. Constance, a 28-year-old divorced mother of one three-year-old child, living at Central Methodist, holds a deep mistrust of South African healthcare providers. After one and a half months in the host country, she has accessed emergency medical care only one time, due to a pregnancy. "I am pregnant. There's no suitable place for me," Constance said, "The other women here said if it [birth] is at night, security will call an ambulance. But there's no transport. For the ambulance to come, you have to have booked a hospital for the birth, so for me it is a problem." Constance then sought assistance from the Catholic Archdiocese of Johannesburg, Ministry of Zimbabwean Immigrants, where she received a letter asking hospital officials to assist Constance in booking a birthing room. But, "They did nothing. I had a letter and they said you had to book with the nearest clinic. They told me, 'We don't assist you foreigners.'" She then sought help at Loveday Hospital, but found that they were on strike for the week. Constance did feel that if she would possess the right immigration (asylum) paperwork, she would have received proper hospital care in South Africa. But for the moment, she admits, "I am not feeling very well here because the situation is not settled for me here. At first I was feeling welcome, but how they treated me in the hospital, I don't feel safe."

The Zimbabwean women also reported suffering racism via the general population as well as from institutionalized workers, clerks, nurses, and doctors in Johannesburg-area hospitals. Jennifer, a 27-year-old single mother of two children, a 10- and a 6-year-old girl, lives at the Central Methodist Mission Church. After three years in South Africa, she has accessed emergency medical care 12 times, primarily due to persistent coughing episodes. Back in 2008, she tried to get medical care for her persistent cough from Hillbrow. At the hospital, she was asked for her asylum papers, which she did not possess. Without the proper immigration papers, they said, "We are not going to help you," she said. She has successfully sought medical care about 10 times at the nearby MSF Clinic, where she said the staff is always friendly and helpful. She has also successfully sought medical care at Loveday clinic, where they gave her treatment and free medication. Jennifer thought that if she would possess the right immigration (asylum) paperwork, she would have received proper hospital care in South Africa. Jennifer explained, "I don't think they like us here, especially Zimbabweans. Some they call at us and shout at us. They call: '*Makwerekwere!*,' '*Makwerekwere!*' They say we are taking their jobs." (The colloquial use of the expression *Makwerekwere* is used by native South Africans as a derogatory term for non-South Africans, or as a disparaging term given to black immigrants from any Africa country outside of South Africa.) Despite these shouted comments, Jennifer said she likes her new home country. "I don't want to go back home, I like South Africa. Maybe I can go to America."

Like Jennifer, Fungayi reported maltreatment by Johannesburg-based healthcare providers. Fungayi, a 22-year-old married woman, has a high school education and currently lives at Central Methodist Mission Church in downtown Johannesburg. During her Zimbabwean-South African border crossing, Fungayi claims she had all of her money stolen from her—taken by a corrupt South African border patrol agent. Fungayi has accessed EMS five times in three months, primarily due to complications with her first pregnancy. The first time she went to Hillbrow seeking medical care, she complained of fever, vomiting, headaches, cough, and body weakness during her pregnancy. Fungayi said the head nurse told her: "You are a Zimbabwean. You must go back. We are sick and tired of Zimbabweans here. You can only come back if there is water or blood." She left without anyone checking her temperature, vital signs, or any fetal monitoring. One month prior to our interview, Fungayi lost her baby. At 6 p.m. on Sunday, July 13, Fungayi had sharp, stabbing abdominal pain and called for an ambulance to come to the church. She and her husband, Ishmael, waited three hours before they decided to take Fungayi to nearby Hillbrow. When she reached Hillbrow, they didn't even attend to me, she said. "We've been attending Zimbabweans all day!" the nurse shouted at Fungayi. The pain was so much, Fungayi said, she finally lay down on the floor. She was crying and writhing in pain and when the staff finally attended to her, they rushed her by ambulance to Johannesburg's main General Hospital. When she arrived at the hospital, six hours after her onset of abdominal pain, she miscarried. At 12 minutes before midnight, the nurse said to me: "Your baby is already dead. Here's your baby. Do you think it's dead?" There was no doctor, just one nurse who came, Fungayi explained. She said that she was torn and need stitches [due to perineal tearing], but wasn't given any pain medication. Ishmael said he felt like the nurses tried to blame him, asking him, "When was your wife's last check-up?" Ishmael and Fungayi were only allowed five minutes to see their first child before the stillborn boy was taken to the morgue. Ishmael, crying and overcome with grief, was told he had to leave because he was "making too much noise." Ishmael said he had just lost his only child and he thought the staff would comfort them, but instead they "left us alone" and didn't offer either of them comfort or counseling. Fungayi then quietly said, "That day was very tough. I don't ever forget that day. They were very cruel to me." The couple still needs 2,800 Rand for the baby's burial, which they need in order to take the baby from the morgue to a burial plot. Already 800 Rand has been donated by family and friends to help defray the burial costs, but Fungayi and Ishmael are still waiting to get their first child out of the city morgue and into a proper burial place.

But during their interviews, three of the Zimbabwean women (Japera, Precious, and Mercy) expressed their desire to return home to Zimbabwe, despite the country's widespread fiscal challenges. Japera is a 28-year-old single mother of a one-year-old boy; she has seven years of formal education and lives at Central Methodist Mission Church in Johannesburg. After six months in South Africa, she has accessed emergency medical care about three times, primarily due to a severe cough with bloody sputum. The first time she sought emergency medical care for probable tuberculosis was at Hillbrow Hospital, where she was turned away and told she should seek help at her nearest clinic. The second time Japera sought and accessed medical care through MSF, where she received 15 paracetamol, or acetaminophen tablets, an over-the-counter pain and fever reducer. The third time she sought medical care was through Loveday and they, again, gave her 20 paracetamol tablets. Japera continues to complain of a severe cough with bloody sputum. "I want to go back to Zimbabwe. I don't want to stay here," she explained, "I don't feel safe here and I am sick every day."

Like Japera, Precious wishes she could return home to Zimbabwe. A 34-year-old married mother of six children, Precious lives at the Central Methodist Mission Church in downtown Johannesburg. After four months in South Africa, she has accessed emergency medical care two times, due to back pain, vaginal bleeding, and a pregnancy. Precious and her children are alone in the country as her husband suffered a broken skull in an attack only after three weeks in South Africa. He has returned to Zimbabwe to seek acute and long-term medical care. During the interview, she was holding a six-day-old baby, born at Hillbrow Hospital, in Johannesburg. Two months ago, at seven months pregnant, Precious said she went to Hillbrow in the hopes of getting treatment for back pain, vaginal bleeding and to register her pregnancy for a hospital delivery. She said she received no medical attention and the staff treated her rudely, and "They told me to go back to Zimbabwe. Everyone says 'go back to Zimbabwe.'" Precious has had trouble sleeping, and with a Grade 7 education from Zimbabwe, complains she cannot find steady work in Johannesburg. Six days ago, she walked to Hillbrow at 5:30 a.m. and delivered her child only one hour later, at 6:30 a.m. By 1 p.m. that same day, she was told to leave the hospital and vacate her hospital bed. They told me: "Go back to Zimbabwe."

Mercy, like Japera and Precious, wants to go back home to Zimbabwe. Mercy is a 27-year-old single mother of one six-year-old girl, and has been very unhappy and frightened in her host country of South Africa. Her two-month stay, she explained, has been fraught with fear, theft, and shake-downs from people within her own migrant community. Within the first three days of her stay in South Africa, all of her clothing and lotion and goods were stolen. Some of the people at the church helped her to get clothing, but others harass her at the Central Methodist Mission for money that she doesn't have: "The security guards chase me outside. They don't treat us nicely and they ask five rand from us to get in. The Bishop [Paul Verryn] is here many times, but the Bishop is not at the gate, so every day they ask us for money when the Bishop isn't there." After two months in South Africa, she has accessed emergency medical care two times, due to a severe cough and then to register her pregnancy for delivery at a hospital or clinic. At the time of the interview, she was five months pregnant: "I feel pain. My stomach feels pain. I have had a baby, but this time it doesn't feel good. I left Zimbabwe to get medical help and money for the baby. But no job . . . just promises." Two weeks ago, she had several severe coughing fits and was told she could get free care at a "Doctors without Borders" (Médecins Sans Frontières) MSF Clinic, which is just around the corner from the church. She said the staff was very friendly to her and that they gave her tablets that helped her within two days of taking the medication. "I went to Hillbrow [Hospital] to register my pregnancy. They said 'is full' and they can't take me here. They did not check the baby . . . I was thinking of going back to Zimbabwe to get care. It will be better because they can't chase me away—In Zimbabwe, it's my country and they just want money." Having completed Form 4 in Zimbabwe, she continues to look for cleaning work or any paid task that would help her buy food for her, and medical care for her unborn child. She exhales deeply: "I'm not happy. I want to go home. I have no money, no job. It would be better to start a business there [Zimbabwe] and stay with my family."

Yet despite their challenges as undocumented females, there were a few Zimbabwean women who had come to fully embrace their new life in South Africa. Maiba was one example of this. She is a 29-year-old widowed mother of two boys (a 10-year-old and 6-year-old), she has seven years of formal education in Zimbabwe, has been widowed seven years, and currently lives at Central Methodist Mission Church. After two years in South Africa, she has accessed medical care about six times, primarily due to her own HIV treatment and care. She said she was given a blood test for HIV back home in Zimbabwe and she was told it was negative. When Maiba was tested in South Africa, her results came back positive and she sought care at Nazareth House, a local Catholic charity owned and run by the Sisters of Nazareth, a Catholic religious order of nuns. Her free care at Nazareth House is only a 15-minute car ride away and consists of one tablet per day. Maiba said the staff at the Nazareth House is always very kind to her and she receives good care when she feels she needs it. "I lack good food. I am poor. No work. One meal a day at the church here," Maiba said with a weak smile. But she is feeling better and more resilient under her supervised health care at Nazareth House: "I feel stronger now. I feel good here in South Africa . . . I am very happy."

Again it should be noted that the information reported by the interviewee on her emergency healthcare services was compiled on an unpaid, anonymous, subjective, and completely voluntary basis. Therefore considerations of voluntary disclosure and personal health privacy issues must be taken into account. It should be resolutely stated that the identification of post-care patients on or near any emergency care center by a researcher (myself included) would be inherently and categorically unethical. To do so would not only exacerbate the patient's traumatic event, expose her to further potential mental hardship, stress or PTSD, and/or exploit her conceivable vulnerabilities (such as suffering from vertigo/nausea or being heavily medicated from ER visit), as well as quash patient privacy considerations and any patient-provider privilege. For instance, it is markedly common for people to suffer from an altered mental status (mental incompetence) after head injuries, fever, infections, or diabetic ketoacidosis, etc., which can all cause confusion, amnesia, defects in judgment, and disruptions in perception, psychomotor skills, behavior, and so on. Plus, the women may still be suffering from shock (low blood pressure/septic shock/anaphylactic shock/cardiogenic shock/hypovolemic shock/neurogenic shock), or too emotionally or physically traumatized from their accident/incident to provide a rational accounting of their care. Additionally, the precedence of the emergency is on urgency of the patient's care and treatment, so any intervention or time loss could cause further harm or an exacerbation of the patient's illness/condition. In the United States, the term "ambulance chaser" has become synonymous with an unethical lawyer, as some unscrupulous attorneys use events such as disasters, personal injury incidents, and motor vehicle accidents (referred to as barratry) to locate potential clients. This practice is prohibited and illegal in the United States and is considered a felony charge punishable by imprisonment over one year in many American states (such as Texas). So to solicit post-care patients on or near any healthcare premises would be categorically unethical and potentially illegal for any legal or healthcare practitioner.

Notably, the interview's contents had several observed limitations and defects, including the frequent disparity between the interview's written level and the respondent's educational level. The overall interview was too brief, so the majority of the interviews readily morphed into personal narratives explained from the woman's own convictions, experiences, perceptions, and of course, subjective viewpoints. Conversely, some of the more positive aspects of the interview were its anonymity, the presence of many open-ended questions, as well as the 'stand alone' ease of the queries, which respondents could choose to answer or delete without affecting the overall results or subsequent questions.

The interviews also had several other significant limitations, including sample size, time since the incident, inherent subjectivity, disclosure (or the avoidance of disclosure) of personal and medical information (such as HIV/AIDs status), the respondent's lack of medical knowledge to ensure proper medical reporting, and translation shortcomings. Translation issues were only apparent in the Mexican interview group, as the entire Zimbabwean interview group possessed a good working knowledge of English. The Zimbabwean interviews were lengthy, polite, and relatively unproblematic. But the Mexican group of women possessed extremely poor English communication skills, with the exception of only two women with whom I could speak with directly (without assistance of a translator). Oftentimes, the Mexican women would voice extensive narratives in Spanish, only to have the translator quip an (perceptibly) much-abridged version of what the woman had attempted to communicate to me. This proved frustrating, as there were numerous times when the English-Spanish-English exchanges broke down when neither the translator nor the interviewee were very certain of English or Spanish medical terminology, body organs, and bodily function/malfunction (such as diarrhea versus bloody bowel movement, or an asthma attack versus respiratory distress, etc.). Moreover than not, some of my interviews with the Mexican women started out as seemingly rudimentary care, but concluded as life-threatening cases of communicable Hepatitis, cancer, and high-risk pregnancies. In many instances, it was only through my medical knowledge of trauma, diseases, drug regimens, quarantine protocols, and conventional medical treatments that I could identify, along with assistance of the woman and the translator, the interviewee's probable diagnosis/condition with their responses. In all refugee or migrant healthcare settings, the proper translation of all health-care communications play a hyper-critical role. Everyone concerned—including the patient, the patient's family or caregiver, healthcare provider, and translator—must understand all relevant patient symptoms, health history, chief current complaint(s), etc. How you tackle this singular (seeminlgy innocuous) challenge can undeniably make or break your patient's successful treatment.

To add to those complexities, international fieldwork involves additional negotiated ethical densities, such as being observant and cognizant to histories of colonialism, development, globalization, and local realities in order to "avoid exploitive research or perpetuation of relations of domination and control" (Sultana 2007, 375). Many scholars like Foucault and Bulter, among others, have noted that power is "both a precondition for constraint of subjectivity" (Burman 2004, 18). Nagar and Geiger claim that existing approaches to self-reflexivity "arises from a failure to distinguish systematically among ethical, ontological, and epistemological aspects of fieldwork dilemmas," and, critically speaking, "does not re-distribute income, gain political rights for the powerless, create housing for the homeless, or improve wealth" (2007, 2–5). Perhaps more significantly, reflexivity does nothing to dissolve the tension between the (inherently and inevitable) hierarchical and inequitable structure(s) between the researcher and the researched group (England 1994). Nagar and Geiger go on to note that while scholars demand ethnographical research to include the researcher's personal discourse on their identity, self-reflexivity, and positionality, no such expectancies or requirements pertains to scholars utilizing quantitative methodologies—which can, in worst-case scenarios, cause a further "marginalization of ethnographic research and personal narratives in producing knowledge" (2007, 5). For the purposes of this research an application for the utilized interview questions was submitted to the University of the Witwatersrand's Human Research Ethics Committee in May of 2010. After the HREC committee's review, seven revisions were identified, and after the revisions were submitted and considered by the HREC Committee, the amended application was approved on August 10, 2010. This particular research involved ethical quandaries such as: How could I locate undocumented women who had sought out (exclusively) emergency care? And how could I acquire these women's contributions when I wasn't paying for their time and interview participation? I felt (very strongly) that publicizing a payment of any amount would bring in a deluge of fictitious experiences from these (often) economically desperate women. So paying them for the re-telling of their experiences was immediately and categorically out of the question. Instead, I attempted to locate these women through trustworthy undocumented acquaintances, who (I hoped) would open the lines of communication through their already established, long-term, trusted, and mutually shared/common experiences and relationship(s). The collection of interviews in Houston proved, very surprisingly, much more difficult to ascertain than the Zimbabwean interviews. First, the Mexican women were more fearful of the American Immigration Naturalization Service's police and so were far more hesitant to speak with anyone who identified them as "undocumented" in the United States. Second, the communication between myself and the Mexican women could only be conducted in Spanish, as only two of the women spoke enough English for me to speak directly with them (and without translation). This was particularly frustrating as some of the 'richness' of these women's experiences were, in a manner of speaking, 'lost in translation'—the lack of depth and intensity of the Mexican women's interviews definitely is illustrated throughout the text of this research. I speak rudimentary Spanish, only recognizing key healthcare phrases (words like sick, vomit, headache, and so on) and some basic expressions—but not enough to grasp the more subtle nuances and emotional state during their experiences. Third, they seemed especially suspicious of my possible motivation(s) for soliciting and collecting this information. For instance, one of the women I interviewed had been diagnosed with a communicable/infectious disease several years ago and was concerned that I was gathering information on her once again. Conversely, the Zimbabwean women were very trusting that we were there to 'help' (even indirectly through academic research) and not 'harm' them (turn them into immigration authorities or the [more feared] police)—yet this tenet did not hold true of the interviewed

Mexican women. Four, the Mexican women were more pressed for time and far less willing to spend time re-telling their experiences.

As with any cross-cultural interview, inherent hierarchical structures, power relations, and positionality were also exerted. As a white Westernized American, viewed also as a healthcare provider and the president of an American NGO (by Zimbabwean women only—Mexican women were not aware of this status), my status was (possibly) more skewed to that of a Western emergency healthcare worker than that of an academic scholar soliciting research. Even though the women were made aware of the doctoral research, I believe it was my status/position as an international humanitarian healthcare/aid provider that most of the women seemed to retain as pertinent to them. I ascertained this through my personal interviews with them, as the vast majority of them perceived me as an "NGO healthfield worker" rather than an academic social scientist. The inequity of the power relations were far more pronounced among the (more) newly migrated Zimbabwean women, as the vast majority of them remained homeless and/or in sub-standard housing in Johannesburg. Despite the Mexican women being more established (on average) in their host nations than their Zimbabwean counterparts, they remained apprehensive and more guarded in their conversations with me.

From my personal feminist perspective, I would prefer to expend (at least) comparable reflexivity energies on what historical, biological, and social experiences bound us—even as obviously diverse and palpably dissimilar as we were from one another—rather than to focus exclusively on the ample (quite incalculable) issues that divided us. So my introspection into self was not only as a 'vulnerable observer' but also as a 'vulnerable participant' through my experiences as a single mother, a wife, a woman, a sister, a first-generation American citizen, a former emergency room patient, and a disaster evacuee. It was indeed these shared/common constructs of trauma, violence, and social power that had provided not only the catalysts, but the very quintessence (i.e. affinity, compassion, and empathy) that propels my disaster aid research and emergency medical service. Yet while reflexivity can make the researcher and the concerned groups more mindful, empathetic, and/or responsive to their asymmetrical (or even exploitive) relationship, it does nothing constructive to rectify, alter, or eliminate these conflicting roles, inequitable power states, and ethical dilemmas.

THEORETICAL RIGHTS VS. PRACTICAL EFFECTS

As the time-worn proverb counsels: *In theory, the difference between theory and practice is small. In practice, the difference between theory and practice is huge*. This research's interviews demonstrated that while theoretical healthcare rights and practical (evidence-based) healthcare rights assert common goals, the reality lies somewhere between the two. Indubitably, theory and evidence are neither irreconcilable nor diametrically opposed, and there are theory-guided evidence-based practices that integrate both approaches successfully, especially in medical practices. But the reality of many forced migrants' experiences in claiming their accorded healthcare rights has proven theoretical, and not practical, in its nature. This holds true with many of the Zimbabwean and Mexican women interviewed for this research as well.

According to the Human Rights Watch report "Neighbors in Need: Zimbabweans Seeking Refuge in South Africa": "Zimbabwean refugees continue to struggle to gain access to emergency and non-emergency health care . . . Despite these theoretical rights, there has been slow progress in giving them practical effect: there is no national or local government policy explicitly reiterating these rights or establishing procedures to help refugees claim them with service providers" (2008, 34). This particular sentiment is evident in the interviewed women, as well as the Zimbabwean refugees I met and worked with over seven years. While the national precedents and laws for emergency and basic health care are theoretically and legally in place in South Africa, the practical effects are of their day-to-day adherence and enforcement are lacking. Some of challenges non-nationals face in accessing health care in South Africa, according to CoRMSA, includes being treated poorly by medical staff or practitioner, language barriers, denial of treatment, and cost issues. But CoRMSA is quick to point out that barriers to health care can differ greatly by area and city—Migrants in Johannesburg experience the highest degree of difficulty, followed by Durban, Cape Town, Pretoria, and Port Elizabeth (2009).

This is an opinion subscribed to by Dr. Gavin Mooney, a professor of Health Economics at the University of Sydney and an Honorary Professor at the University of Cape Town. Mooney wrote a startlingly candid piece on healthcare ethics for the Johannesburg-based *Saturday Star* on April 7, 2012. The tenacious article was entitled: "Something is Rotten in SA Hospitals . . . NHI Will Fix It," and it painfully ripped off the Band-Aid of the festering sore of inequity in healthcare expenditures. He wrote of the ethics of equality in healthcare access and other "social determinants of health" as indicated by the Green Paper by National Health Institute, a paper that reported that half of the SA healthcare expenditure goes to 16% of the population; the other half to 84% (Mooney 2012). "In terms of health care, apartheid is alive and well," Professor Mooney writes, but he also struggled with the ethical dilemma of an economist debating ethical quandaries noting that it is when people "move from efficiency to equity" that the ethical questions become much more problematical for a society and that "there are limits to what any society can spend on health and health care and that is true of all countries whether rich like the U.S. or a middle-income country like South Africa" (Mooney 2012, 15).

An example of this is Gladys—turned away from life-saving oncological (cancer) treatment in Houston, Texas, because she was not a United States citizen and couldn't afford private insurance, or health care. Gladys, a 19-year-old mother of two, said she had to return back home to Mexico, where she is a citizen, in order to afford life-saving medical treatment for thyroid cancer. Gladys reported that in 2010, she went to a downtown Houston-area emergency room for severe pain and swelling in her throat: "They were nice and good to me. I still talk to the nurse from there. But the treatment was too much money and I had to go back to Mexico . . . It is difficult to get treatment in this country because it is expensive." Gladys received a successful treatment for her condition back in Mexico and has since returned back to the United States. "The dentists are even too expensive here. So, I had to just have the teeth pulled out," she said. Gladys noted that she is depressed and sad, and she continues to worry about her undocumented immigration status in the United States.

Yet in all fairness, there are irrefutable differences in EMS care in South Africa and the U.S.A. As one example, South African EMS providers have to absorb the costs involved in the transport of non-insured patient's care. EMS personnel in South Africa are required to meet the standards of the governing body, the Health Professions Council of South Africa (HPCSA). Reported response times of 15 to 20 minutes for P1 (Red/Critical) calls in urban areas are considered acceptable, while in rural areas, response times of up to 40 minutes to an hour, (for similar calls) are not uncommon, according to unofficial blogs by South African paramedics. In fact, on June 8, 2013, the world's media reported that the ailing 94-year-old Nelson Mandela was picked up in an ambulance that broke down en route to from Johannesburg to the Medi-Clinic Heart Hospital in Pretoria. The BBC News reported that Mandela had to wait 40 minutes in freezing winter temperatures before the transfer to another ambulance took place (BBC 2013).

Another example of South Africa's flawed EMS service was uncovered in Anale's interview, as a 28-year-old single unmarried mother of one child, living at Central Methodist. Anale has accessed emergency medical two times in the two years she has been in South Africa, once for an injury and once for a pregnancy. She explained that she's here in Johannesburg with five other members of her family, but without the baby's father, as he left when she was seven months pregnant. Anale said that when she was five months pregnant she sought to register her child's birth at the local area hospital. They asked her if she was Zimbabwean and, when she responded "yes," they told her to "come back later." This past week Anale had the harrowing experience of calling for EMS and not receiving any help. At midnight this past Saturday night, Anale went into labor and an ambulance was called to the church. The women who were helping her waited and waited, calling the service several times to check on the ambulance's progress. Finally, after waiting three hours for an ambulance, at 3 a.m. she gave birth to the baby in the women's cramped, soiled upstairs toilet at the church: "The ambulance never came. I took a taxi cab to the hospital." At 7 a.m., Anale was finally taken with her new baby boy to the General Hospital in Johannesburg for a check-up. She now has a job as a housekeeper that pays 1,000 Rand a month and is adjusting to her new life in South Africa well. "I don't want help. I want more hope. I want to help myself," summarized Anale.

Contrariwise, in the United States, most EMS services run on some (or all) public funding. Some American ambulance services are operated by the city (municipal department, local, regional or state governments), a hospital, or a private company. Municipalities can fund their EMS via property taxes and service fees, and many small communities staff their EMS through volunteer corps of workers. It is exceedingly common for local residents to train and voluntarily staff their local EMS and/or fire corps without any salary or pay—even in larger U.S. cities. Third-party providers (private; for profit; fee-for-service) ambulances are becoming more and more common in America these days. These EMS crews and ambulances can be contracted by small communities or local hospitals, elderly care centers, companies, or other entities. This option can reduce response time, and increase resources and staffing expertise in specific skill sets (extraction, high-rise, hazardous materials, ski rescue, water rescue, etc.). Many EMS workers are "dual-qualified" as firefighters and EMS corps members, doubling their usefulness and knowledge in traffic accidents, and utilizing their time more optimally for both medical and fire emergency calls. Cities can require their third-party/hired services to maximum response times, usually between 10 to 15 minutes. It should be noted that an "ideal" response time for EMS is eight minutes or less, especially in cases of cardiac arrest (when a patient's heart stops beating and blood stops circulating oxygen through the body). In cardiac arrest, the patient's lack of oxygen will damage the brain irreversibly, making survival impossible. According to the *Journal of the American Medical Association*, every minute of untreated ventricular fibrillation—or cardiac arrest—leads to a reduction in survival of up to 10% (Valenzuela et al. 1992). That being said, the survival of (out-of-hospital) cardiac arrest patients was significantly higher if: CPR is initiated by Basic Life Support (BLS) level co-responders within four minutes of the initial call for help, and paramedic-level Advanced Life Support (ALS) care is on-scene within eight minutes (Valenzuela et al. 1992). (Response time can be defined as the interval between the time the patient's location, callback number, and patient complaint are known, and the time the ambulance EMS crew arrives on scene.) When both of these conditions were present, the study reported a 43% survival rate. Hence, these types of findings have helped to create the eight-minute EMS 'Gold Standard' among ambulance services. Of course, problematic factors such as high total call volume, call-volume density, traffic congestion, poor road maps and signage, and other geographic factors (frontier regions, rural communities, suburban areas, etc.) can make it arduous to maintain the eight-minute response-time standard. These outlying areas can implement air ambulance or helicopter services, or create first responder (with minimal first aid, CPR, AED and emergency childbirth training) community programs.

In conclusion, this chapter has attempted to lay the groundwork for future gender-disaggregated healthcare research, thereby assisting emergency healthcare planners and providers to more effectively and successfully plan for women in future forced migrations, emergency healthcare events, and disasters. This research's interviews queried six dimensions of each woman's emergency healthcare experience and provided firsthand accounts (Voices of the Women) with both direct and indirect quotes from the women obtained during their one-on-one interviews. In the end, what the interviews uncovered was the gaping chasm between theoretical healthcare rights and the practical effects of those rights. Most notably, in America the Mexican women could ill afford sky-high medical costs and this undermined their trust in the all-too profitable 'business' side of America's 'wallet biopsy' defensive health care—constructing rarely insurmountable fiscal barriers to health care. Meanwhile, in South Africa, the Zimbabwean women's experiences uncovered blatant xenophobic denials of care combined with a deep mistrust of the country's medical institutions and personnel—constructing physical and psychological barriers to health care. Hence, the day-to-day reality of many forced migrants' experiences in claiming their accorded healthcare rights has proven to be more theoretical than practical in its distribution and disposition.

Chapter 5

Host Country Health Care

"There are too many of them . . ." exhaled the distraught South African nurse over the daily influx of Zimbabwean refugees into her Johannesburg-based hospital. In those six words, the nurse had succinctly characterized the rampant 'them' versus 'us' mindset within national institutions that serve to form, foster, and feed the fertile ground for engendered and institutionalized 'fear of foreigners.' The application of social justice shapes the tangible foundation of public health care, and it is well within the realm of each nation's policy makers and healthcare institution's procedures to resolve either to passively 'cultivate' or to actively 'eradicate' the structural violence of xenophobia.

In this chapter, we will start our initial analysis by taking an overarching 'national view' of the core concepts, functions, primary goals, and evaluations that can set up the parameters for these two host countries' healthcare systems. We will delve into those parameters, as well as determinants and injustices within these public healthcare systems, plus federally mandated patient rights, and American and South African Constitutional provisions for healthcare access. What follows is an assessment of federally mandated public health responsibilities and the rights to private personal health can run a contentious race—and how infectious diseases are no respecters of national perimeters and can flow unimpeded across manmade borders via exposed populations. The current battles waged by both South African and American healthcare systems against infectious/communicable HIV/AIDS, cholera, measles, tuberculosis, multi-drug resistant tuberculosis (MDR-TB), and extensively drug-resistant tuberculosis (XDR-TB) etc. will be addressed. Then roles of each host country's EMS 'gatekeeper' to care, triage, will be reviewed. The similarities and differences between American and South African triage indexes will be explored, compared, and explained. Then fiscal sustainability of both countries' current state of intense medical inflation of public and private healthcare system costs—considering the rate of influx of undocumented patients, staffing shortages, and America's 'anchor baby' inflow which automatically sanctions U.S. birthing citizenship—will be reviewed. "Why should anyone care?" looks at how the overcrowding of both host country's Emergency Departments (ED) can lead to patient's prolonged pain and suffering, adverse patient diagnosis, medical errors and patient outcomes, increased total patient length of stay in hospital, increased ambulance transport times for patients, and even death. Finally we will take a look forward and report on the current state of American and South African healthcare reform, including 'Obamacare' in the U.S.A. and South Africa's emergency care boost from reforms and some national 2010 FIFA World Cup EMS initiatives.

A TALE OF TWO HOST NATIONS' HEALTHCARE SYSTEMS

To begin our look at national public and private healthcare systems in South Africa and the U.S.A., it is beneficial to first note the core concepts, functions, and goals that set the parameters for these systems. Within the realm of national public health care is emergency healthcare, and by law, most healthcare professionals are bound by their public oaths of service to provide lifesaving treatment. Critical emergency healthcare treatment is often regarded as a basic global human right, regardless of whether the individual has a means to pay for treatment. This remains a core universal component and conviction in emergency, or lifesaving, healthcare services. In its most fundamental form, the three core primary goals for health systems, according to the World Health Organization, are set forth as good health, responsiveness to the expectation of the population, and fair financial contribution . . . and that health systems are not just concerned with improving people's health, but with protecting them against the financial cost of illness (2000). The WHO's right to health mandate contains the four so-called AAAQ elements, which include availability, accessibility (non-discrimination and physical, economical and informational accessibility), acceptability (medical ethics and cultural- and gender-sensitive), and quality (2000). Health systems can promote or violate human rights to health care in their design and implementation and vulnerabilities to poor health can be reduced by following the WHO's steps to respect, protect, and fulfill people's rights to healthcare systems. Going one step further, Duckett (2004) proposed a simplified two-dimensional approach in how to begin to evaluate healthcare systems: quality, efficiency, and acceptability on one dimension, and equity on another. Clearly, any investigations that uncover, evaluate, and prevent inequities in healthcare systems remain as critical components and benchmarks in a nation's system surveillance.

But inequities in healthcare systems and services do exist, and they often disguise themselves as poor physical, economical, or informational accessibility, inequitable treatment, discrimination, or inadequate or disrespectful provider response and treatment. Ethicists like J.A. Rawls contend that inequity in health care is an acute social injustice, as poor health profoundly limits opportunities in employment, relationships, and social and political participation throughout a person's lifecycle (1971). Yet how each society views its own fairness and injustices in public health care is very "reflective of the society's willingness to tolerate very large inequalities of income, wealth, and economic and political power" and the "more unequal a society is in economic terms, the more likely it is to be in terms of health care" (Geiger 2006, 208). While the provision of public health care remains a significant challenge, the health care of refugee and forced migration populations pose an even more taxing challenge, with its mix of codependent and conflicting political, social, fiscal, gender, and human justice issues. According to Toole:

> One of the most stark examples of the relationship among social justice, inequality and poor health outcomes occurs among populations that are forcibly displaced . . . It is the poor and powerless who are eventually faced with no option other than to flee their home and sometimes their country to survive. The toll on the health of displaced populations is severe. (2006, 190–203)

Drawing on Krieger's ecosocial theory that the proposition of social justice is the foundation of public health care (2006), it is imperative that any possible social inequalities in health be researched, documented, evaluated, monitored, and addressed. According to the World Health Organization, health policies can promote or violate human rights, and the right to health contains the four primary elements of availability, accessibility, acceptability, and quality (2007). Like all human rights, the right to health imposes obligations of respect, protection, and fulfillment, but draws distinctions between a party's *inability* and/or *unwillingness* to comply with its health obligations (WHO 2007). (Based on the previous propositions from Krieger and the World Health Organization, the rationale for studying these issues at this time include the need to address social justice, gender justice, and human rights abuses in emergency healthcare access among female refugee/forced migrants and gender-disaggregated healthcare data by social advantage that is neither maternal-nor familial-based). Therefore it is imperative to research, clarify, and develop some of the theoretical framework which can address social and gender-based injustices in refugee/forced migrant health care. According to Krieger, there are four components in addressing social injustices in health care, including: theory, which is research "used to explain, and guide research on and take actions to address inequalities in health";

monitoring, which documents these inequalities, especially whether or not they are increasing or decreasing; etiology, which tests hypotheses about the causes of these inequalities in the population distribution of some health statuses (like disease, death, disabilities, etc.) and the access and provision of appropriate health care; and prevention, which develops, evaluates, and improves methods to assess efforts to address these inequalities as well as the adverse consequences of poor policies and programs (2006, 463). This research primarily focuses on research and some preventive measures and recommendations that can be used to improve efforts to address inequalities in female forced migrants and undocumented refugees' emergency health care. Krieger also notes that context, time, and place, and its attention to political, economic, social and cultural (i.e. gender-based), physical, ecological, public health, and medical factors all help define the "model of determinants of public health" (2006, 464).

According to the WHO in 2007 the global expenditure for healthcare costs was in excess of $4.1 trillion (USD), about a per-person average of $639. But each nation's healthcare expenditure varies widely: with a high of $6,037 in the U.S.A. (Kaiser 2007), to $221 in South Africa (2001), to $491 in Mexico, and finally in Zimbabwe, $139. Current doctor-to-patient ratios stand at 1:8,000, considering that the World Health Organizations' 'world standard' is set at 1:500 (WHO 2004). Accordingly, the WHO draws direct and significant correlations between wealth and health expenditure on populations, with reports showing that "increasing health expenditures are associated with better health outcomes especially for low-income countries" (WHO 2010).

So to begin, when we review South Africa's public healthcare system we see that parallel public and private systems coexist. While the public system serves the bulk of its population, it has been (historically speaking) chronically underfunded and understaffed, and this division may continue to perpetuate racial inequalities created in the Apartheid era of the twentieth century. According to South Africa's Human Sciences Research Council, the nation spends 3% of its GDP and just over 15% of government expenditure on health care. Government health expenditure accounts for 45% of the total health spending, and the remainder is financed from private sources (health insurance and out-of-pocket expenditure), with total health spending equaling 7.5% of GDP (Martin 2003). In South Africa, suitable public health care is a government-supported mandate, and each province has its own healthcare department. According to the Constitution of the Republic of South Africa Act No. 108 of 1996, South African law clearly defines the right of access to healthcare services as guaranteed by law. The Department of Health in South Africa is "committed to upholding, promoting and protecting this right and therefore proclaims this Patient's Rights Charter, also known as the Patient's Health Charter, as a common standard for achieving the realisation of this right" (Appendix C) (1997, 1). There are 12 primary areas covered by this rights declaration, including: a healthy and safe environment; participation in decision-making in the development of health policies and on matters affecting their health; access to health care (including timely emergency care, regardless of one's ability to pay; provisions for special needs in the case of newborn infants, children, pregnant women, the aged, disabled persons, patients in pain, HIV or AIDS patients; counseling without discrimination; palliative care; a positive disposition displayed by healthcare workers that demonstrates courtesy, human dignity, patience, empathy and tolerance); knowledge of one's health insurance/medical aid scheme; choice of health services; treatment by a named/identified healthcare provider; confidentiality and privacy; informed consent; refusal of treatment; a second opinion; non-abandonment/ continuity of care; and complaint resolution. Other provisions also include forms of fee-based healthcare and basic education. In other words, undocumented Zimbabweans in South Africa have a legal right to emergency and basic healthcare and primary education, but no rights to social assistance or a valid work permit. The exception to these rules is for asylum seekers, who are granted rights to study and work (Human Rights Watch 2008). South Africans or undocumented residents without insurance may avail themselves of care at local area clinics, NGO clinics, or public hospitals.

Conversely, it is interesting to note that in America there are many constitutional provisions for public education, but there is no explicit constitutional right to shelter—or health care. The United States is the "only advanced industrial nation with the absence of a universal healthcare system," legal rights to health care, and a government-led social responsibility platform in health (Freedman 2006, 486). In the U.S.A. the share of GDP devoted to health grew from 8.8% of GDP in 1980 to 15.2% of GDP in 2003 (Kaiser 2007). This almost seven percentage-point increase in the health share of GDP is larger than increases seen in most other high-income countries. Yet care in the U.S. does have significant portions of publicly funded insurance and networked health hospitals. For instance, Medicare offers assistance to the elderly and disabled, Medicaid serves some of the poorest populations, and state-run insurance policies covers children of low-income families. Medicaid is a large provider and is a federal/state funded program that provides emergency and necessary health care to low-income families, pregnant women, elderly people, and those with disabilities and dependent children and related caregivers. The Veterans Health Administration offers low-cost health care to U.S. military veterans through a large nationwide network of government hospitals, and retired or active duty personnel and their dependents can receive benefits through TRICARE coverage. (See 'Major U.S. Government-Sponsored Programs and their Availability to Undocumented Immigrants,' Figure 5.1.)

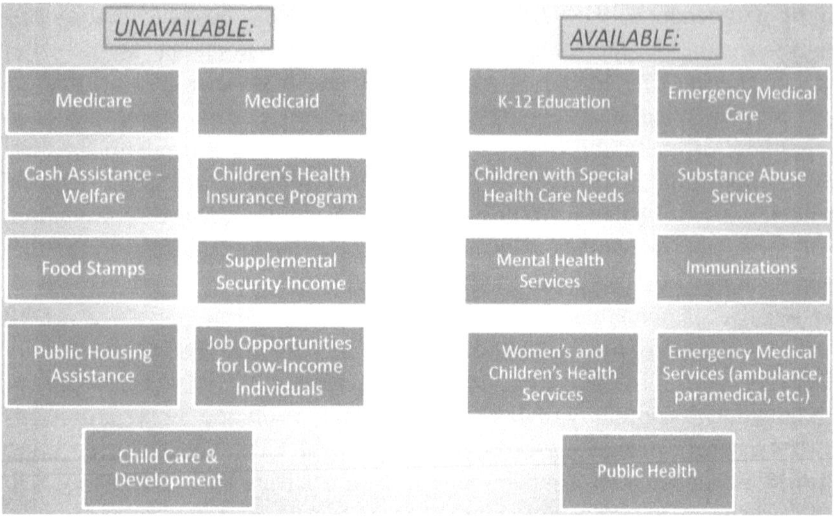

Figure 5.1 Major U.S. Government-Sponsored Programs and their Availability to Undocumented Immigrants

In comparing a patient's constitutional right to healthcare access, two more dissimilar countries that the U.S.A. and South Africa would be challenging to find. But there are some American federal laws ensuring quality care and emergency care for citizens and undocumented migrants, some of which include: the Emergency Medical Treatment and Active Labor Act (EMTALA), the American Medical Association's "Patient's Bill of Rights," and the Consumer Bill of Rights and Responsibilities (adopted by the U.S. Commission on Consumer Protection and Quality in the Health Care Industry in 1998), and more. The benchmark 1999 American Medical Association's Patient's Bill of Rights includes the statement that patients have a "right to essential health care" and covers six primary rights: the right to considerate and respectful care; the right to obtain a complete current information concerning his diagnosis, treatment, and prognosis in terms that the patient can understand; except in emergencies, the right to receive information necessary to give informed consent prior to the start of any procedure and/or treatment; the right to refuse treatment; the right to every consideration of the patient's privacy; and the right to available adequate health care. The sixth principle allows for access to emergency services so that if any person—citizen, out-of-country visitor or undocumented migrant alike—has severe pain, injury or sudden illness, they have the right to be screened (triage) and stabilized utilizing emergency services. The person also has the right to access these services without needing to wait for authorization (insurance, immigration paperwork, proof of payment, etc.) and without financial penalty. (See Department of Health & Human Services Fact Sheet on the 111-page bill in Appendix E.) While there are other pieces of federal legislation that impact patient and/or hospital care, a landmark bill that specifically covers emergency healthcare facilities and patient emergency treatment was passed 13 years earlier in 1986, aptly dubbed the "Patient Anti-Dumping Law" (Appendix F). This U.S. federally mandated "EMTALA," also known as COBRA (the Consolidated Omnibus Budget Reconciliation Act of 1986) or the Patient Anti-Dumping Law, was passed in 1986 and requires every ED operating in the U.S.A. to treat anyone who enters with an "emergency" to be treated. EMTALA is a federal statutory-regulatory complex, consisting of statutes (legislation passed by U.S. Congress) and regulations (mandates approved and adopted by the U.S. Centers for Medicare and Medicaid Services, a division of the Department of HHS, to enforce and further define the EMTALA statute 42) (USC 1395dd, part of the U.S. Code). Whether or not an individual is insured, able to pay for medical services, or an undocumented immigrant—they must be screened and treated until discharge or stabilized for transfer to another hospital or facility. These are some of the decisive and indispensable legislation that insure both documented and undocumented patients receive access to emergency services—including proper screening at triage, stabilization, or treatment—regardless of their ability to pay or proof of citizenship. These mandates directly assist in addressing the uneasy nexus between patient's rights to personal privacy and overarching good of public health welfare, defined as "The science and practice of protecting and improving the health of a community, as by preventive medicine, health education, control of communicable diseases, application of sanitary measures, and monitoring of environmental hazards" by the American Heritage Dictionary (2013). It is this precarious teeter-tooter of private rights versus public welfare accountabilities that we will address next.

PUBLIC HEALTH ETHICS

The current global blight of infectious disease—in the form of HIV/AIDS, Ebola, cholera, and malaria—illustrates how infectious diseases are no respecters of national perimeters and can flow unimpeded across manmade borders via exposed populations. In broad-based medical terms, infectious diseases, also sometimes referred to as communicable or transmissible diseases, are spread through a variety of conduits and activities. Airborne respiratory diseases (like tuberculosis), vector-borne (mechanical or biological), and gastrointestinal diseases (like cholera) can spread rapidly through such pedestrian and unintentional public acts as coughing, sneezing, talking, drinking from contaminated water or food sources, and even via contaminated inanimate objects. Sexually transmitted infectious diseases (like HIV/AIDS) are transmitted via sexual intercourse or acquired through contact with bodily fluids, such as blood or needle transmission. Other infectious diseases, like malaria, dengue fever, and viral encephalitis, are carried and transmitted by flies, mosquitoes, fleas, and other arthropods. People, objects, insects, and animals can transmit these often rather preventable diseases and the result of widespread transmissions can lead to an epidemic, which affects a disproportionately large group of individuals within a population, community or region, or even a pandemic which affects human population across a large region, continent, or global arena. The most recent pandemics include the HIV pandemic, 2009 avian flu, and 2014–2015 Ebola pandemic. Because undocumented immigrants do not undergo federally mandated medical screening (unlike those who may be admitted for legal residency), there has been a resurgence of previously nearly eradicated and/or long extinct diseases into some countries' public health system. Overall some of the infectious diseases that pose a public health risk and are suddenly seeing a marked climb in transmission rates in developed countries in recent years include tuberculosis, leprosy, dengue fever, whooping cough, cysticercosis (parasitic disease from pork tapeworm), polio, Hepatitis A, B, and C, Ebola, and more.

The worldwide epidemic of the human immunodeficiency virus (HIV) and acquired immunodeficiency syndrome (AIDS) has placed severe hardships on displaced persons as well as the refugees' 'receiving states' due to the onus of the disease's transmission, long-term care, social stigmatization, and pandemic nature. Making matters worse, the HIV/AIDS epidemic has been ubiquitous with negative stereotypes, misinformation, misconceptions, and social taboos and stigmatization. AIDS stigma and discrimination can take the form of prejudice, ridicule, abuse, and maltreatment, including but not limited to, poor treatment in healthcare facilities, psychological damage, erosion of rights, as well as an apprehension among potentially infected individuals to seek testing and treatment. Based on a wide range of data, including household and antenatal studies, the UNAIDS/WHO reported in July 2008 that South Africa had 5.7 million people estimated to be living with HIV, one of the highest rate in any single country, with a 18.1% adult prevalence of those aged 15–49 years at the end of 2007, with high and low estimates at 15.4% and 20.9%. (Refer to Chart 5.2 'Adult HIV/AIDS Rate Comparison in Mexico, South Africa, U.S.A., and Zimbabwe.') Among females, HIV prevalence is highest among 25 to 29-year-old women. As for the Zimbabwean populous, it follows closely behind South Africa with 15.3%. Conversely, in the U.S.A., the prevalence rate of HIV/AIDS among adults is 0.6%, or a low and a high estimate from 0.4% to 1%. As for the Mexican populous, it ranks

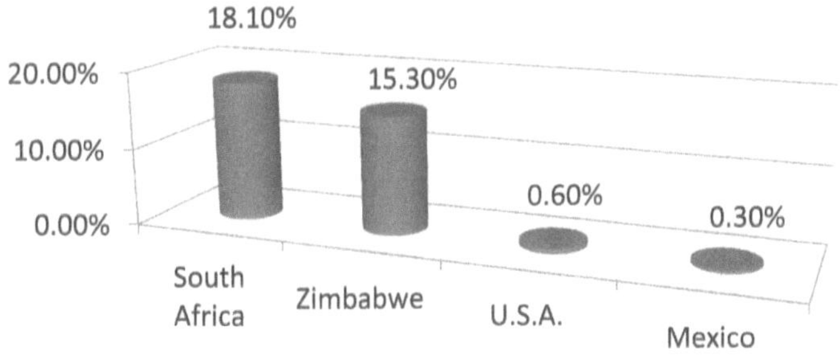

Figure 5.2 Adult HIV/AIDS Infection Rate Comparison in Mexico, South Africa, U.S.A., and Zimbabwe 2008

the lowest in our research group of four countries, with an HIV/AIDS infection rate at 0.3% (UNAIDS/WHO 2008).

In the U.S.A. the number of AIDS cases has remained stable since the 1990s, and in 2007 a 69% drop was reported in AIDS-related deaths (since 1994) (UNAIDS/WHO 2008). In the U.S.A., HIV is not even among the top 15 leading causes of death, and mortality rates from AIDS-related causes in 2007 alone dramatically dropped 10% in a single year, yet the costs of antiretroviral (ARV) prescriptions remains at average annual cost of $20,000 (CDC, 2015). But a non-citizen's access to in-country/host nation ARV treatment can vary greatly, dependent upon a nation's income level, national and local healthcare laws and access policies, transportation, residential area, logistical and social restrictions, etc. For instance, free antiretroviral treatment (ART) access for non-nationals in South Africa, according Joanna Vearey's "Migration, Access to ART and Survivalist Livelihood Strategies in Johannesburg" research, "reflected both the gendered nature of the disease and the gendered patterns of health-seeking behavior" in that one-third of the respondents were male and two-thirds were female (2008, 368). She also found that access to ART allowed the migrant women to maintain or regain their survivalist livelihood, depending upon when the treatment was initiated.

So what might be some of the causes behind tuberculosis as the leading cause of death in South Africa in 2010? In truth, the nomenclature "cause of death" assigned to some mortality cases can be somewhat misleading and even lead to various misrepresentations. For instance, we know that HIV weakens a person's immune system, allowing other diseases (like tuberculosis) to affect and eventually kill the patient. But the "cause of death" classification attributed and reported to such a case will be TB, not HIV, as the disease which caused the patient to die. But the initial infection of HIV/AIDS should not go unreported, or at least reported as a contributory factor—a comorbid disease (pertaining to a disease or other pathological process that occurs simultaneously with another) in many of these scantily reported global medical mortality and morbidity reports.

Yet another alarming public health risk in South Africa is the current growth of multi-drug resistant tuberculosis (known as MDR-TB) and extensively drug-resistant tuberculosis (known as XDR-TB) in the country's provinces. Drug-resistant forms of tuberculosis, both XDR-TB and MDR-TB, are ravaging HIV and other immuno-compromised populations. Since PPD (purified protein derivative) TB testing doesn't seek the *Mycobacterium tuberculosis*, but rather only tests if the patient's immune system is combating the bacteria—many HIV patients lack sufficient immune activity to either fight the infection or properly respond as "positive" to the PPD test (AIDSMEDS 2012). Therefore, perfunctory TB testing is not as dependable in HIV-positive people with compromised immune systems, so many times a diagnosis of TB will not be made until (further) acute symptoms arise, and/or more sophisticated testing like X-rays, sputum, or blood tests are performed.

In Paul Farmer's *Infections and Inequalities: The Modern Plagues* book, he cited five assertions that "hold true" for drug-resistant tuberculosis as well as global HIV strategies: effective treatment cannot be solely the province of wealthy countries, as TB remains, along with AIDS, the "leading infectious cause of adult death in the world today"; cost-effectiveness cannot be the only measure by which public health interventions are evaluated as any costly intervention that serves destitute and sickly populations is diametrically opposed to profit-making corporate welfare goals; research in developing countries has to include social justice initiatives because, as Farmer notes, "poor people are excellent lab rats but unlikely patients" concerning first-world diagnostics on third-world data collection subjects; more effective prevention strategies are needed as the "education as the only vaccine" tactic is "nether accurate nor wise"; the notion of 'limited resources' should not be silently accepted as verbatim now. Farmer insists that there is no data to prove that there are currently scarcer fiscal resources available today, when there are more, not less, effective therapies for diseases than ever before (1999, xxiii–xxvi). Clearly, greater and more equitable access to effective medical services and treatments is a necessary first step in staunching these life-threatening national and global infectious disease epidemics.

Due to its high prevalence of HIV/AIDS patients, South Africa has taken many measures to bring about successful local treatment programs and 'down referrals' that allow for patients to receive ARV at the primary local clinic level (sometimes referred to as a 'medical home'), thereby relieving ED and district hospitals of some of the burden of the initiation and continued distribution of medications and checkups. For instance, the Eshowe Hospital and two feeder primary clinics in Uthungulu District (Kwazulu

Natal) used a rapid cycle improvement methodology to return stable patients on ARVs to their local PHCs for chronic care via an eight-step process that transitions the site of care, and incorporates all stakeholders such as clinic teams, pharmacies, ARV clinics, and patients. The results of the 2006 referral program was a 10% decrease of the chronic care burden at the district hospital level and an increase of 56 stable ARV patients referred back to a primary setting over a period of 8 weeks (IHI 2007). It is through innovative practices like the aforementioned program in Kwazulu Natal that countries could improve their provision of HIV services to the ever-growing populations of migrants and citizens who must receive lifesaving ARV medications and treatment.

In a textbook example of yet another infectious disease spreading unchecked across borders—the cholera outbreak in August 2008 spread into nine neighboring countries of Angola, Botswana, Malawi, Mozambique, Namibia, South Africa, Swaziland, Zambia, and Zimbabwe. During this pandemic, the numbers of cases of cholera were estimated at over 155,708, with over 4,686 resulting in mortalities (UNOCHA 2009). To date, every province (10 out of 10) in Zimbabwe has been affected, case fatality rates remained unacceptably high, and after an initial downtick in 2009, the spread of the disease seems again to be on the rise. In a report on December 8, 2008, UK Prime Minister Gordon Brown said, "This is now an international rather than a national emergency. International because disease crosses borders," Brown added, "International because the systems of government in Zimbabwe are now broken. There is no state capable or willing of protecting its people" (CNN 2008). In a benchmark regional response, the United Nations Office for the Coordination of Humanitarian Affairs, UNICEF, the World Health Organization, other regional NGOs, policy makers, and healthcare providers from the nine affected countries gathered in February 2009 in Johannesburg to hold a workshop aimed at strengthening cholera response. Migration and other compounding factors such as adequate sanitation, political instability, chronic food insecurity and lack of safe drinking water were all identified as contributing factors to the cholera outbreak (UNOCHA 2009). In the 2014 and 2015, we were to again see these contributing factors during the Ebola pandemic that began in December 2013 in Guinea near the border with Liberia and Sierra Leone. As of July 5, 2015, some 27,609 cases and 11,261 deaths have been reported worldwide, with the mortalities in these same three countries, as reported by the Data Team at *The Economist* (2015).

At its nucleus, the Ebola and cholera pandemics are rather classic 'global textbook' cases of why countries bordering such infectious disease epidemics must address efficient prevention and treatment in areas that lack effective domestic healthcare policies and access. Today more than ever, there is an unquestionable link between public health and reported (documented) and unreported (undocumented) mass human mobility that cannot be ignored. Due to the continued displacement and mass international and cross-border migration patterns, diseases that used to be a confined to the parameters of a 'national emergency' have grown into a burgeoning multinational crisis. In the current global environ, when we choose to ignore our neighbor's contagious communicable disease it can plot an inexorable, and potentially fatal, path. It is these public health and welfare choices, medical programs and parameters—such as an EDs triage algorithm—set by emergency healthcare providers and planners, governments, and hospital systems that play a pivotal role in the equitable and effective dispensation of public health care.

However, we cannot begin to discuss healthcare systems and poor health outcomes in emergency medical medicine without first addressing the far-reaching 'gatekeeper' mechanism for all Emergency Room care: Triage. This is the overriding 'directive' that all emergency care facilities and providers obey; therefore, it must be defined, clarified, and extensively addressed for the purposes of this study. If we do not understand what mandates allow or disallow for emergency service interventions, how can we begin to address any deficiencies in care?

The purpose of EDs triage protocols and triage personnel is to prioritize incoming patients by the acuity of their injury and illness and to rapidly and accurately identify the small percentage of patients requiring immediate care and/or life-saving interventions. It is here that the reader should note that it is this all-important triage mechanism that assesses and classifies the undocumented females within our research as an 'emergency' (oftentimes free treatment) or 'non-emergency' (perhaps no treatment offered) patient. It is precisely this reason why triage becomes the critical 'gatekeeper' mechanism for the screening of all Emergency Room patients.

At this time, we should also note the critical legal and medical service distinction between 'emergent/emergency,' 'elective,' 'non-emergency,' and 'chronic' (long-term) assessment in triage, and how that affects a patient's receipt of care by the host country's healthcare institution. As an example, a positive HIV/AIDS individual can present with nothing more than the flu (influenza) or a broken leg at an ED, and have no outward evidence of the disease. So the more urgent problem for this patient would be the detection of the disease and the limiting of the transmission through diagnosis, information, and behavior modification. But the mere presence of HIV/AIDS in the patient, without any life-threatening complications (such as pneumonia, central nervous system infections or malnutrition), may not be considered an 'emergency' condition requiring care in the ED. HIV/AIDS is a chronic, long-term progressive illness that can warrant ARV (anti-retroviral medicines) and treatment over many years. In other words, HIV/AIDS can be likened to diseases such as diabetes and hypertension (high blood pressure), in that there can be complications (such as ketoacidosis, strokes, heart attacks, etc.) from the disease itself that would illicit emergency treatment from an ED, yet the mere presence of the disease itself is not considered a life-threatening emergency event.

As EDs in both the U.S.A. and South Africa struggle to cope with overcrowding and the influx of unrecognized immigrants, there is a critical need for an equitable, medically valid, and reliable triage acuity rating system in order to sort these incoming patients more rapidly and accurately. For example, in the United States, the vast majority of emergency room physicians normally use a three- or five-tier nationally recognized triage index. The commonly used three-level scale includes these acuity levels: emergent (or emergency), urgent, and non-urgent (ENA 1997). Patients are rated as emergency (or emergent) if they have a problem that poses an immediate life or limb threat. Patients considered 'urgent' are those that require prompt care, but can wait up to several hours if necessary. 'Non-urgent' patients have conditions that need attention, but time is not a critical factor (ENA 2001). The five-level ED triage algorithm, called the Emergency Severity Index (ESI), provides clinically relevant stratification of patients into five groups from ESI-Level 1 (most urgent) to ESI-Level 5 (least urgent) on the basis of acuity and resource needs (ESI 2008). The ESI-Level-1 patient presents to the ED with an unstable condition and could die without immediate care. They are seen immediately because timeliness of interventions can affect morbidity and mortality. Some examples of ESI-Level 1 patient symptoms and vital signs include cardiac or respiratory arrest, severe respiratory distress (such as agonal respirations), a pulse oximetry (SpO_2) reading of <90, a critically injured trauma patient who presents unresponsive, severe bradycardia or tachycardia with signs of hypoperfusion, anaphylactic reaction, a baby that is flaccid, or hypoglycemia with a change in mental status (ESI 2008). On the other end of the urgent spectrum are Level 4 and Level 5 patients, who from a clinical standpoint can wait several hours to be seen by a doctor or a midlevel Physician's Assistant, perhaps through an available 'fast-track' venue that can handle low-acuity patient assessment and/or treatment.

Conversely, due in part to its low 1:8 doctor to nurse ratio, South Africa has developed a nurse-based Cape Triage system through the universities of Cape Town and Stellenbosch (Cape Triage Group 2005), but no formal triage system is in place and uniformly applied throughout the country. The Cape Triage was implemented in January 2006 for ED and pre-hospital/paramedic use, scoring patients in three categories (adult, pediatric, and infant) using a very exact and rather complex Triage Early Warning Score (TEWS) scoring system and five triage color codes (red, orange, yellow, green, and blue) (Cape Triage Group 2005). In fact, in a three-month implementation of the

Cape Triage system at the 200-bed acute care GF Jooste public hospital in Cape Town, South Africa, showed a rather significant drop in ED wait times, from 237 to 146 minutes (Bruijns et al. 2008).

Triage systems encompass trauma and medical cases and ideally it can process patients more quickly, decrease wait time and the ER congestion, determine appropriate treatment area in the ED, and also provide a good 'continuity of care' between the pre-hospital EMS and ED departments. But it is imperative that healthcare providers uniformly follow prescribed acuity levels in triage and that these acuity parameters are precise, clinically accurate, and medically relevant enough to ensure equitable treatment. Yet the mere provision of care parameters does not automatically ensure the proper observation of the acuity parameters, so they must also be uniformly enforced. Clearly it is within these critical "life-and-death" parameters that emergency healthcare decisions for undocumented women are being made—and it is these policies, and the people, doctors, hospital systems, and governments that create them, that must be the focus for addressing each country's current state of politics and policies in undocumented and forced migrant emergency health care.

CODE BLUE: SUSTAINABILITY OF CURRENT HEALTHCARE SYSTEMS

The sustainability of both countries' current healthcare financing policies is at risk, and particularly in the U.S.A., issues with finding financing could be the load that tips many U.S. hospitals into bankruptcy. By any measure, the U.S. healthcare system is the most expensive in the world, whether viewed as health expenditures per capita/person or on total expenditures as a percent of GDP. The excessively high costs in U.S. health care can be attributed to several core issues including the costs of modern medical technologies, prescription drugs, the growth of for-profit hospitals, an aging population, uninsured patients (15% on average), and soaring administrative costs (19.3%–24.1%) due to complex multiple payer systems, according to a University of Maine report aptly named: "The U.S. Healthcare System: The Best in the World or Just the Most Expensive?" (2001).

Yet there continues to be a marked upsurge in global healthcare costs. For example, in the U.S.A. (which has had both a high level of health spending per capita and a high rate of growth in that spending), the share of GDP devoted to health grew from 8.8% in 1980 to 15.2% in 2003 (Kaiser 2007). This almost seven percentage-point increase in the health share of GDP is larger than increases seen in other high-income countries. Conversely, South Africa's spending in 2005 was 7.7% of GDP, with 40% of funding flowing through its public care system, which serves some 80% of population, and 60% into the private sector (Harrison 2007).

Currently, according to the Centers for Medicare and Medicaid Services, the federal government in the U.S.A. provides $250 million a year to reimburse states for emergency health care for patients without immigration documents (Preston 2006). Two-thirds of the money is distributed based on the estimated number of illegal immigrants in a state, while the remaining one-third of the funds is given to the six states where the majority of illegal immigrants are seized (CMMS 2006). In order to help reimburse these "top six" states, the U.S. federal government paid the state of California $66.6 million, Arizona was reimbursed $47.7 million, Texas was given $47 million, New York was paid $12.2 million, Illinois was reimbursed over $10 million, and Florida was given $8.7 million (CMMS 2006).

Yet within the U.S.A., many public hospitals are left to struggle with uneasy ethical decisions: Demand immigration documents and deny care to any patient who cannot produce them, or provide unrestricted public healthcare access to any patient in need of care. As examples, two large public hospitals in Texas, each chose different paths to public healthcare access. Parkland Hospital in Dallas, Texas, offers low-cost care to low-income patients—without any immigration registration or paperwork. But JPS Health Network in Fort Worth, Texas, demands that any non-U.S. citizen provide legal immigration paperwork in order to receive financial assistance in nonemergencies, such as routine and elective surgeries and treatment of illnesses (Preston 2006).

As for women, female patients that are pregnant constitute a large group of undocumented immigrant patients in Texas, and with good reason: Texas hospitals get so-named 'anchor babies,' children of women who run across the Mexico-Texas border to give birth to a baby born on U.S. soil, and who immediately become a U.S. citizen. According to the *NY Times*, Parkland Memorial Hospital in Dallas, Texas, delivered 11,500 babies in 2005 to mothers who were probably illegal immigrants, comprising approximately 60%–70% of its entire maternity ward operation (Preston 2006). Estimates are that between 300,000 and 350,000 "anchor babies" become citizens of the U.S. as mandated under the nation's Fourteenth Amendment to the U.S. Constitution: "All persons born or naturalized in the United States, and subject to the jurisdiction thereof, are citizens of the United States and the State wherein they reside" (Cosman 2005, 7).

By comparison, the sustainability for the current financing and subsistence of the South African healthcare system is under attack, with some reports putting the nation's yearly medical inflation as high as 25% (Pallot 2010). The South African healthcare system also struggles, as the American system, with people who lack insurance and overcrowded emergency departments or government-run health institutions, which are far cheaper but tend to lack trained staff, space, drugs, and equipment. Like America, only one in five South Africans has private medical insurance (Pallot 2010). In an astonishing twist, South Africa flows 40% of its funding into its public care system, which serves some 80% of population, and 60% into the private sector (Harrison 2007). The rather posh private healthcare sector in South Africa is something to boast about. With some 200 state-of-the-art private hospitals—similar to numbers in to the United Kingdom—even the singular spending on per-patient medication in the private sector is 13 times higher than in the state system. Yet four in five people in South Africa cannot afford to use their services. So the vast majority of South Africans, asylum seekers, and undocumented Zimbabweans are cared for within the primary care system that has no hypercritical shortage of well-qualified medical staff, unlike many of its African neighboring countries. The bulk of the estimated three to four million Zimbabweans in South Africa can also seek free medical care at local Médecins Sans Frontières (MSF) and NGO-run clinics and state-run EDs. In June 2009, amidst numerous xenophobic attacks in the country, MSF clinics reported treating between 4,000 and 5,000 Zimbabweans monthly. The Médecins Sans Frontières June 2009 report "No Refuge, Access Denied: Medical and Humanitarian Needs of Zimbabweans in South Africa" also stated that incidents of injured Zimbabweans being turned away by hospital staff, nurses not tending to 'foreigners,' and rape victims being denied follow-up medical treatment were cited. But Zimbabwean refugees are left few alternatives for care. While some private hospitals in Zimbabwe are still open and maintained, they are fiscally out of reach for average citizens. As an example, a pregnant woman would be expected to reportedly pay out over $3,500 for local gynecologists, pediatricians and anesthetists, in addition to funding her own food, medication, and accommodation for both mother and child—while in South Africa, she might pay less than $70 for all the services up to delivery.

In the same report, the international relief NGO warned that the adoption of a more 'liberal immigration policy' for Zimbabweans was placing greater burdens on South Africa's already stretched healthcare system: "Consultations in our Johannesburg clinic have almost tripled in the last year, a telling sign of the extent to which Zimbabweans are consistently denied access to even the most basic healthcare services necessary for their survival," stated Eric Goemaere, Medical Coordinator at MSF in South Africa (MSF 2009, 1). So the struggle to keep up with increasing numbers of patients in EDs and clinics puts more and more financial, administrative, and staffing strain on already overburdened and understaffed system resources.

Aside from forced migration issues, current economic downturns in South Africa and the U.S.A. are driving more and more patients to emergency departments in their hour of need, which may be accelerated by job and insurance losses, as well as household budget cuts. Why should we care? Accordingly, EDs tend to serve as a healthcare safety net for everyone, the insured and uninsured alike, and their role in both South African and American healthcare systems has never been more critical.

In the U.S.A., EDs serve 120 million patients annually (about half of all hospital admissions), and while ER demand increased 32% over the past decade, the number of EDs decreased by 5% in the past 10 years due to closings and bankruptcies—resulting in higher demands with fewer resources (ACEP 2009). The American College of Emergency Physicians (ACEP) also noted that people age 65 and older represent the fastest growing segment of the population in the U.S. and the group whose visits to the ED are increasing the fastest (2009). These are also the patients who require the most acute care and are admitted to the hospital from the ED most often, factors which could lead to catastrophic crowding in the ED in just a few years. Due to the overcrowded state of emergency rooms, the average wait time in an ER of 3.2 hours can seem interminable. Average wait times in U.S. ER's was 6.2 hours, with seniors waiting an average of 10.6 hours, and patients with incomes less than $20,000 waiting 13.3 hours (Time 2004), but there have been unofficial reports of wait times of over 35 hours in public hospitals in the Los Angeles area.

So what is the impact of ED overcrowding on patient care? According to a 2008 U.S. study from the ACEP Boarding Task Force, overcrowding can cause a wide variety of consequences, including, but not limited to: (1) sick people wait too long for emergency care—ACEP found that more than 10% of patients judged to be "critical" by a triage nurse can wait more than one hour to see a physician. Since early medical intervention leads to better outcomes, delays in patient care can lead to disabilities, increased complications (one study showed patients with acute coronary syndrome had a 6% complication rate in crowded EDs compared to an average rate of 3%), and even death; (2) prolonged pain and suffering; (3) long emergency room waits, and consequently "walkouts" that may need care; (4) increased transport times for ambulance patients—one-third of U.S. hospitals have experienced ambulance "diversion"; (5) increased total patient length of stay in hospital—usually adding on one full day to a stay compared to patients with similar illnesses that were promptly taken into inpatient care; (6) increase in medical negligence lawsuits—the frequency of medical liability lawsuits is increased by a factor of five simply based on whether a patient waits less than 30 minutes to be seen by a physician; (7) adverse events and errors (including medical errors); and (8) finally, in the worst-case scenario, patient mortality. Put succinctly, what causes ED overcrowding can be lack of staffing, hospital overcrowding, lack of proper funding for equipment, staff and supplies, along with a myriad of other administrative and medical care issues.

Perhaps one of the most telling and widely publicized editorials on the myriad of financial and structural challenges facing America's healthcare system comes from "How American Health Care Killed My Father" written by David Goldhill. After the death of his father due to an infection from a well-regarded private hospital, Goldhill wrote an attention-grabbing editorial on the state of the American healthcare system in September 2009 in *The Atlantic*, a major conservative finance magazine. While Goldhill applauded the hard work and efforts of the well-trained medical staff and facilities, he issued a scathing attack on the crumbling core structural concepts, subsidies, and incentives at play in the system:

> All of the actors in health care—from doctors to insurers to pharmaceutical companies—work in a heavily regulated, massively subsidized industry full of structural distortions and that America has built a healthcare system with incentives that inexorably generate terrible and perverse results. Incentives that emphasize health care over any other aspect of health and well-being. That emphasize treatment over prevention. That disguise true costs. That favor complexity, and discourage transparent competition based on price or quality. That result in a generational pyramid scheme rather than sustainable financing. And that, most importantly, remove consumers from our irreplaceable role as the ultimate ensurer of value. (2009, 1)

Goldhill's comments favoring both reform and open market supply-and-demand schematics have been added to decades of rather verbal criticism of a broken system that is in dire need of advanced life support. In recent years there have been marked and widely publicized and criticized pushes for American healthcare reform. Most notably, on March 23, 2010, U.S. President Barack Obama enacted the most expansive social legislation in the United States in decades—the Patient Protection and Affordable Care Act of 2010 (Appendix E). The law did not come into full effect until 2014, and the legislation extended coverage to 95% of Americans, bringing in the estimated 32 million Americans who lack insurance due to costs, some (un-insurable) pre-existing condition(s), or by choice, according to CBS News' "Political Hotsheet" (Jackson et al. 2010). The Hotsheet also reported that illegal immigrants were not allowed to buy health insurance in the state-run exchanges, even if they paid fully for the coverage out of their funds. As for the new legislation's coverage of undocumented immigrants, President Obama declared at a 2009 White House congressional session: "Now, there are also those who claim that our reform efforts would insure illegal immigrants. This, too, is false. The reforms I am proposing would not apply to those who are here illegally" (2009, 1).

Other key components of Obamacare healthcare reform mandates that most U.S. citizens and legal residents have minimal essential coverage for themselves and their dependents, which they can get through their employer, or if their employer doesn't offer health insurance, they can buy it through new marketplace 'exchanges.' For people who decide not to follow the new law, tax penalties began in 2014 and are fully phased in by the year 2016. Reportedly, fines would start at $695 for each uninsured family member, up to a maximum of $2,085, or 2.5% of household income, whichever is greater. One of the precepts of Obamacare was ensuring coverage of preventive and necessary services for women, eradicating gender discrimination by health insurance companies, and making health insurance more accessible and affordable for women and their families. This nation-wide fight was dubbed "The War on Women" and many Democrats and Republicans faced their female constituents in the elections accordingly. According to the United States' American Civil Liberties Union:

> The 'War on Women' describes legislative and rhetorical attacks on women and women's rights taking place across the nation. It includes a wide-range of policy efforts designed to place restrictions on women's health care and erode protections for women and their families. Examples at the state and federal level have included restricting contraception; cutting off funding for Planned Parenthood; state-mandated, medically unnecessary ultrasounds; abortion taxes; abortion waiting periods; forcing women to tell their employers why they want birth control, and prohibiting insurance companies from including abortion coverage in their policies. (ACLU 2013)

Conversely, South Africa has also been making big pushes recently for healthcare-related reform. On World AIDS day in December 2009, Zuma declared a new "era of openness" in the country with the world's largest HIV-infected populous, vowing to extend free antiretroviral drugs in 2010 to HIV-positive infants under one, as well as pregnant women and patients with low T-cell counts who suffer from tuberculosis and AIDS. *The New York Times* reported that Zuma said that 73% of South Africans with HIV also have TB, and the nation will increase state-sponsored ARV drug access to patients with CD4 count at 350 or less—whereas previously the state-sponsored treatment was available only when a patient's CD4 count fell below 200 (Dugger 2010). In May 2010, several media reports cited thousands of South Africans who got tested for HIV and received 100 free condoms each at the launch of the HIV Counselling and Testing (HCT) Campaign. Dubbed the "most ambitious HIV testing campaign in the world," according to SA National AIDS Council (SANAC) co-chairperson Mark Heywood, the HCT "I Am Responsible" campaign conducted free tests on patients at the entry points in all health institutions and hopes to get up to 15 million people tested by

June 2011, aiming to reduce the rate of HIV infection by 50% by 2011 and to provide treatment to up to 80% of affected people, according to an April 28, 2010, report from BuaNews. These remarks and nationwide campaigns are a radical break from former president Thabo Mbeki's very public denial of the HIV threat. In 2006 Zuma was charged with rape, and during the trial he acknowledged that he did not use a condom during sex with a woman he knew to be HIV positive but said he took a shower afterward in the hope of reducing the infection risk. He was later acquitted. As a leader and a Zulu (South Africa's largest ethnic group and one that had abandoned circumcision in the nineteenth century), Zuma said that he had been circumcised and encourages other men to undergo the procedure, which can reduce a man's risk of contracting HIV by more than half.

Additionally, in preparation for the onslaught of tourists for the 2010 FIFA World Cup, South Africa provinces added numerous additional ambulance and health crews to handle the influx of thousands of tourists. For example, the Western Cape Department of Transport donated over 71 new ambulances to the Health Department, which now can boast an available deployment of 130 ambulances, and a goal priority call response time of 15 minutes in urban areas and an hour in rural areas, reported BuaNews on March 24, 2010. South Africa's World Cup spectators could also download the free, brand-new iPhone's "iTriage" application which included healthcare facility mapping and GPS locations of private hospitals in the eight provinces that tourists visited, according to Colorado, U.S.A.-based Healthhagen, the application's creator.

In conclusion, it is imperative that healthcare providers uniformly follow prescribed acuity levels in triage and that these acuity parameters are precise, clinically accurate, medically relevant, and uniformly enforced enough to ensure equitable treatment for documented and undocumented patients. It is within these critical 'life-and-death' parameters that emergency healthcare decisions for forced migrants' and refugees' treatment are being made—It is these policies, and the hospital systems, provinces, and governments that create them that must be a 'principal starting point' for addressing each country's current state of politics and policies in unrecognized migrant emergency health care. While America struggles to put into play its first-ever available universal healthcare system, it continues to offer no explicit constitutional right to health care, and allows each public hospital to struggle with the uneasy ethical decisions of demanding immigration documents (and deny care to any patient who cannot produce them), or to provide unrestricted public healthcare access to any patient in need of care. As the most expensive in the world, the U.S. healthcare system must review and rein in its excessively high costs so that its modern medical technologies, prescription drugs, the growth of for-profit hospitals, an ever-aging population, uninsured patients, and astronomical administrative costs can exist within its complexity of multi-tiered payer systems. All the while, the core composition of American emergency care system remains one of the few rather efficient and more cost-effective sectors, representing a tiny fraction (about 3%) of the $1.5 trillion that the nation spends on health care overall.

In comparison, in South Africa health care is acutely divided along public and private sector lines—with the gaping chasm between the two patently extensive and incontrovertible to any keen observer's eye. What personally was most interesting to note is the extremely high standard of care in public sector hospitals—having personally toured and observed an ED in action in Johannesburg, a facility where the state-of-art equipment, high level of care and staff training was comparable to and/or even exceeded European and American facilities and/or healthcare standards. But it also easy to conceptualize that better pay and working conditions all-too-easily pilfers good doctors and nurses to private hospitals and away from the public sector where they are most needed. The South African Constitution guarantees access to health care and other essential services to refugees, asylum-seekers, citizens and migrants, all regardless of legal status. However, in practice, fears of arrest, deportation, and xenophobia, and a general lack of healthcare rights continue to keep many Zimbabweans from accessing these services. This research and MSF testify to the fact that all too often Zimbabweans are charged exorbitant fees to access public facilities (despite public policies to the contrary), turned away from hospitals when they need admission, discharged prematurely, or subjected to harsh treatment by health staff in the public services. Thus, how each nation views its own equity and justice in public health care reflects the society's tolerance of inequalities of power. Clearly, the more financially, socially, and gender-equitable a society is, the more likely its healthcare system will demonstrate equity. And while the provision of public/universal health care remains a significant national challenge for both the U.S.A. and South Africa, the health care of refugee and forced migration women opens a veritable Pandora's Box of conflicting political, social, fiscal, gender, and human justice issues that politicians, governments, and healthcare providers must wrestle to bring under control.

Chapter 6

Women's Health

In broad-based biological terms, women suffer from many of the same diseases and illnesses as men—but they endure them uniquely as women within their unique physiological and psychosocial variations and contexts. Current research points to increasing exposures and losses in disasters, forced migration, and refugee emergencies, with impacts becoming demonstrably more pronounced due to ongoing social, political, and economic issues that dramatically and adversely affect women's health care. Thus it is imperative that this research address women's very unique medical needs by delving into some of the specific sex-based biological differences in disease, treatment, and care (pain, patient assessment, and mental health) experiences of these women. The purpose of this chapter is to explain the biological variations in women's physiological composition, thereby delineating the link between the biological and social vulnerabilities of women in disaster and refugee situations.

PATHOLOGY AND PHYSIOLOGY OF WOMEN'S HEALTH AND DISEASE

According to Adar and Stevens, while women are affected by many of the same health concerns as men, the conditions "manifest and are experienced differently . . . The prevalence among women of poverty and economic dependence, their experience of violence, negative attitudes towards women and girls, discrimination due to race and other forms of discrimination, and a lack of influence in decision-making are social realities which have an adverse impact on women's health" (2002, 162). Echoing the importance of studying sex-based health differences is a watershed 2001 American

Institute of Medicine report which asserted that "studying sex differences, like other biological variations, can yield greater insight into understanding biological disease mechanisms, leading, in turn, to improved treatments and outcomes" (Levy and Sidel 2005, 77). The study of more effective treatments and outcomes among female refugees and forced migrants, like Mexican and Zimbabwean women, form a crucial dimension to addressing women's health needs in their host and home countries. A relative newcomer on the scene in medical sciences is gender-based biology, a science that can trace its conceptual launch back to the late 1980s. This intriguing, but fledgling arena of science identifies "physiological, cellular, tissue, organ, and system level and the effects of pharmaceutical agents on males and females" (Langley 2003, p. ix). To begin a look at gender-based biology, several ubiquitous points can be made in male-to-female biological variations. For instance, from a universally focused view, women tend to suffer from more illness, nearly always suffering more disease and utilizing more health services than men (Langley 2003, p. x).

Pharmacological and toxicological differences on how the sexes respond to medications or environmental agents are probably much more significant than is conventionally recognized or acknowledged. Even the half-life and clearance of a drug can differ considerably when administered to a male or female. Awareness of these biological differences is vital in both the triage and treatment of healthcare patients in post-disaster settings. Anatomic and physiological reasons for these differences include factors that can affect the absorption, distribution, and metabolism such as gut transit times (44.8 hours in men and a much longer 91.7 hours in women), total body water (42 liters in men and only 29 liters in women), gastric acid pH (1.92 in men versus 2.59 in women), and body fat percentages (21% in men to 32% in women) (Langley 2003). When you analyze these variances, you can ascertain that a woman, on average, has 40% less body water than the average man, and men also have a higher basal metabolic rate. All of these factors interact to make women's absorption and metabolism of drugs exceedingly dissimilar from that of men. For example, since a woman's body content of fat is higher than a man's, drugs that are fat soluble will be stored in the fatty tissue. Toxins and drugs stored in the fat persist longer in the body. Of particular consequence is that women have more cycles of fat loss and gain due to dieting and pregnancy, therefore toxins stored in the fat may be released during these cycles, causing the onset of various disease(s) (Langley 2003). Moreover, there are also biological disparities in the behaviors of certain detoxifying enzymes in the liver which are affected by male and female hormones, so overall "women tend to have greater bioavailability and slower clearance of drugs compared to men, the consequence being that the correct dose for males may be relatively high for females" (Langley 2003, 308).

An intriguing piece of research in 2008 by Chloe Bird and Patricia Rieker is found in their book *Gender and Health: Constrained Choices and Social Policies*, wherein the authors acknowledge that socioeconomic health disparities contribute to, and interact with, gender differences. But the authors go one step further to include the differences in the lives of men and women and their physiology—they also account for factors other than inequality of resources, discrimination, and other unfair or prejudicial treatment. Within their construction of the well-known and so-called 'morbidity/mortality paradox'—whereby women live longer than men yet have higher morbidity (illness) rates—Bird and Rieker astutely adopted to include other innate biological forces and external individual choices, such as national health policies, community actions, work, family, personal choices (to smoke or not to smoke cigarettes for example), and biological processes. This they dubbed as their 'Conceptualization of Constrained Choices' (see Figure 6.1) which duly places national policies at the apex of the constrained choice diagram in that a country's policies creates priorities and establishes procedures for the society's provision of healthcare entitlements and rights. These critical policy choices could prove more economical and "lessen the disease burden and spiraling costs associated with the large aging population confronting virtually every country" (Bird and Rieker 2008, 244).

As for general life expectancy, it is critical to take into consideration the average expected lifespan of both a forced migrant's home and host nation into account before drawing excessive or generalized conclusions on healthcare issues. For instance, among both male and female populations, the

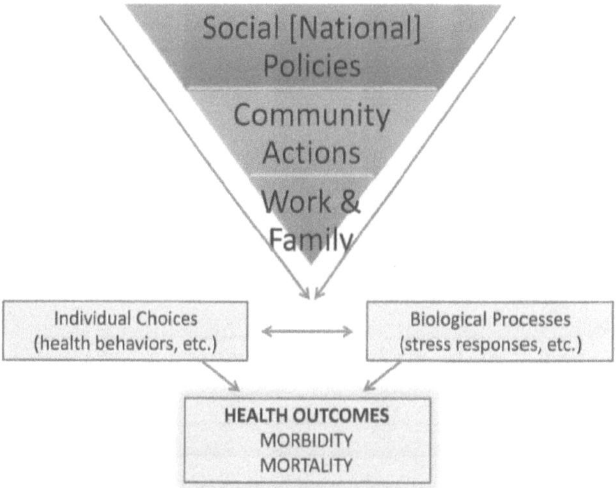

Figure 6.1 Conceptualization of Constrained Choice

average life expectancy in the U.S.A. sits currently at 78.24 (ranked 49th worldwide), followed by Mexico at 76.16 years (ranking 71st), South Africa at 49.10 years (215th worldwide rank), and finally Zimbabwe at 47.55 years (219th worldwide ranking) (CIA 2010). For a longer-range comparison over that past four decades from 1960 to 2008, see figure with World Bank World Development Index data, Figure 6.2.

From a gender perspective, in the United States the average life expectancy in 2008 among men was approximately 75.29 years and 81.13 years among women, and in Mexico the average life expectancy among men was approximately 73.5 years and 78.78 among women—but conversely, in South Africa the average life expectancy among men was 49.63 years and women 48.15 years, and in Zimbabwe, men's expectancy was 45.08 years and women 43.46 years (CIA 2010). The male-female life expectancy gender reversal from the U.S.A.-Mexico to South Africa-Zimbabwe can be explained through a number of studies. The trend for increased longevity among women tends to be a rather universal tendency. However, many studies point out that the greater the socioeconomic affluence of a nation, the greater is the disparity in male to female life expectancy rates, with female rates remaining higher. In countries that are less affluent, the female advantage in life expectancy tends to narrow, according to the WHO (2010). World Health Organization studies show consistently that as countries get richer, male mortality tends to decline less than female mortality, as women are generally more health conscious in rising economies and men have much higher smoking rates, poorer diets, and exercise less (2000). But according to a 2009 report by the South African Institute of Race Relations

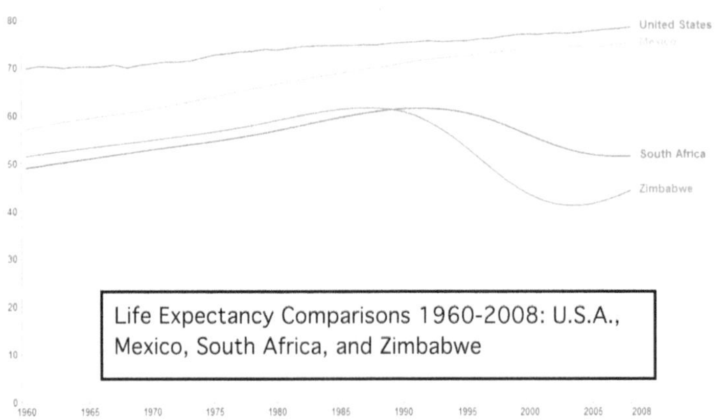

Figure 6.2 Life Expectancy Comparisons 1960–2008: U.S.A., Mexico, South Africa, and Zimbabwe

(SAIRR), South Africans are dying younger and in increasing numbers, with HIV/AIDS to blame. The report also noted that South Africa is one of only six developing/developed countries where life expectancy fell between 1990 and 2007, with only Zimbabwe showing a steeper decline (SAIRR 2009).

Some of the other gender-specific and sex-based based pathologies and physiologies in women's health and disease that will be explored in this chapter include women's unique experiences with the physical and psychological effects of transition in forced migration; sex differences in migration patterns; pregnancy complications; and some heightened risks and differing clinical manifestations of PTSD and rape. From our research of undocumented Mexican migrants in the U.S.A. and forced Zimbabwean migrants in South Africa, we will study the various types of emergency health services utilized, real and/or perceived barriers to healthcare services, rates of depression, as well as the variation of the acuity (the level of severity) and infectious nature of the women's reported illnesses. This research will elucidate the need for disaster planners, aid agencies, and healthcare providers to decrease post-disaster/forced migration emergency healthcare costs, alleviate unnecessary suffering, and successfully reduce female, infant, and maternal morbidity and mortality by meeting women's physiological and psychological needs in a more proactive, efficacious, and gender-aware manner.

According to migration researchers Bhugra and Jones (2001), a woman's migratory process can be split into three marked stages: pre-migration, when she plans and decides on the move and still has access to healthcare services and pre-existing health status; migration and physical transition, when she moves into host society; and finally, post-migration, when the woman deals with the new society, learns new roles, and how and where to access healthcare services. All the while, there are many socially based issues like identity, social unity, organization, and interaction that come into play within the host and migrant communities. Other mitigating factors that can readily be linked to a migrant's health in their host society can also include any pre-existing health conditions (illnesses, trauma, disabilities, known and unknown diseases, injuries, etc.), exposure to health risks in their pre-displacement location, and prior access to health services in their native country.

When it comes to sex differences in migration patterns, men are predominant. For instance, there is a strong pattern of male migration of Zimbabweans into Johannesburg, with ratios of 63% male to 37% female reports (Vearey 2008). In this, you'll note that among Zimbabweans migrating into Johannesburg, South Africa, 63% were male and only 37% were female, and correspondingly the number of male to female Mexican migrants into the United States was 55.8% (male) to 44.2% (female). In both the Mexican and Zimbabwean populations' comparison, men were the predominant sex among migrant communities. As for sex differences in Mexican migration into the United States, again men remain predominant.

It is noteworthy to report that in South Africa the annual adult (male and female) mortality rates for short-term returning migrants are generally 1.1 to 1.9 times higher than those of residents and long-term returning migrants (Collinson et al. 2009). So clearly there are adverse factors at work, such as stressors, poor health care, and other mitigating causes that are affecting and stunting the average life expectancy of short-term returning migrants in South Africa. What also seems to hold true, generally speaking, among sex differences in migration patterns is that while there may be a lower migration rate, the female rates of stay in host countries are longer. According to LatapÍ and Martin, male migration often prevails because having "a wife at home is cost-efficient, conforms to gender norms, and also enables men to move back and forth without losing standing in village and kinship structures" (2008, 18). For example, according to the same aforementioned researcher's report, once Mexican women leave they are more likely to stay in the United States, and when women leave Mexico the entire household migrates, especially since female migrants tend to be younger, less mobile, and more dependent on social networks and family ties than men (only 7% female-led household reported).

FEMALE MIGRANTS AND EMERGENCY CARE

Even in countries like South Africa and the United States that provide emergency healthcare services and access, female Zimbabwean and Mexican migrants can fail to benefit from these services for a variety of reasons. Language barriers, illiteracy, and poor communication between migrants and the host nation's healthcare providers are certainly observable causes (and of course not the exclusive domain of women). But how women in the migrant and forced migrant communities perceive their health and their decision-making power to affect it are prominent variables. Undocumented female migrants can harbor fear, superstition, dread, and gross misperceptions about immigration risks and emergency provisions in the host countries' healthcare system and resort to accessing health care only in dire, life-threatening circumstances. Logistical issues such as a lack of transportation, funds, or knowledge of local area healthcare facilities and providers can also be barriers to migrants' effective healthcare access. So when host countries fail to empower female migrant communities with the knowledge of their legal rights to emergency health care, it is akin to relinquishing the migrant's right to health care at all.

Our research showed significant variances in the 10 Mexican and 14 Zimbabwean woman's real or perceived barriers to seeking emergency health care—with the vast majority of the woman's reported barriers serving as telltale indications of the current issues faced by these undocumented populations in the host countries of South Africa and the United States. Our use of the terms "real or perceived barriers" bifurcates her obstacles, if any, to emergency health care as actual (as in fact-based), or as assumed (or suspected) barriers, which may be asserted and presumed as truthful by the woman, but remain unproven in its circumstance. The women were allowed to declare none, one, or more than one barrier out of a list of choices, but they were also encouraged to augment or construct their own barrier choices. Of the women's perceived and real barriers to access emergency health care, only immigration status and lack of funds were noted as shared obstacles between the two groups of both the Mexican and Zimbabwean women. Of particular note was that among the interviewed 14 Zimbabwean women, their fear and distrust of local healthcare providers and facilities was their top apprehension in seeking health care. Even before lack of funds or their undocumented immigration status, these Zimbabwean women mistrusted and were keenly suspicious of the care and treatment from South African healthcare professionals. Their evident and observable mistrust of healthcare personnel and authority figures may well have been fostered to some extent by their reported previous negative encounters with police, border guards, immigration, and other government/authority representatives (as noted in the complete transcripts of the interviews). Several of the women explained having been sexually assaulted, robbed, and/or physically threatened by Zimbabwean and South African border guards, immigration officials, and police officers in uniform. One such report came from Fungayi, a 22-year-old interviewed Zimbabwean woman, who said she had all of her money stolen from her, taken by a dishonest South African border patrol agent during her crossing at the Zimbabwean-South African border. In Johannesburg, Fungayi miscarried her first baby at a local public hospital named Hillbrow (Hillbrow Hospital is about a 30–40 minute walk from the Central Methodist Church) reporting how nurses had shouted at her to leave the emergency room and "Go back to Zimbabwe," refusing to help her even though she was in terrible pain and about to miscarry. "That day was very tough. I don't ever forget that day. They were very cruel to me," Fungayi said.

And Fungayi is not alone. Five out of 14 Zimbabwean women reported being fearful and having little to no trust in healthcare providers in South Africa. This trepidation and distrust of South African nurses, doctors, and healthcare providers was the top obstacle reported by undocumented Zimbabwean women seeking emergency health care. Most of the woman reported extremely negative past experiences from South African public hospitals, and only the women who had sought out healthcare services from Médecins Sans Frontières (Doctors without Borders) or other NGOs reported that were satisfied and that they had been equitably and respectfully treated by healthcare providers. One of our surveyed Zimbabwean woman, a 23-year-old mother, explained that when she and her baby were ill, both Joubert Park Municipal Clinic and Hillbrow Hospital in Johannesburg, turned them away at the waiting room, refusing to provide even primary triage or treatment for either. But when she approached the local MSF Clinic, she said she and her child were treated with kindness and given free medication. The young mother explained that she is now "scared of the government" and no longer trusts hospitals in South Africa.

The secondary concern, or barrier, of our interviewed Zimbabwean women to access emergency health care was a lack of funds to pay for any services, supplies, or medications. Mercy, a 27-year-old Zimbabwean mother of one, stated that she "went to Hillbrow [Hospital] to register my pregnancy. They said 'is full' and they can't take me here. They did not check the baby . . . I was thinking of going back to Zimbabwe to get care. It will be better because they can't chase me away . . . In Zimbabwe, it's my country and they just want money." Lastly and equally reported by two women each was their undocumented immigration status as a barrier to seeking emergency health care, and "no barriers" were reported by the two women during the interview.

Among our 10 interviewed undocumented Mexican women, overwhelmingly their top barrier to emergency health care—reported by 8 Latinas—was their undocumented immigration status. Mary, a 38-year-old mother of three living in Houston, said: "You need a Gold Card or legal documents for everything here." The Gold Card she is referring to is a Harris County (Houston) Hospital District that offers financial assistance for medical care to low income individuals and families. If eligible, candidates receive this discount to cover medical services at county clinics and hospitals at nominal to free costs for care. Another 42-year-old Mexican woman noted: "Because of my immigration status I couldn't get the Gold Card . . . I couldn't speak English and no one told me what happened to me. I felt like I was lost. They said I owe $5,000. I couldn't think of what I would do to pay the money."

The undocumented Mexican women's secondary reported obstruction was money, with several citing huge upfront sums in the tens of thousands of dollars for an elective (non-emergency) surgery or treatment for a diagnosed cancer. One of the interviewed women who reported being quoted a significant upfront fee was Zoila, a 43-year-old married mother of four children, living in suburban area surrounding Houston. She called the UTMB, whose patient intake staffer told her she needed to bring in a minimum of $25,000 U.S. dollars before they would take her as a patient for gynecological surgery. But she also added that she has no fear of American hospitals or doctors, "I love the United States and they give you a lot of things. I feel free to ask for help. The doctor is a doctor and not the government." Many of the Mexican women said that any medical or even dental treatment in the United States was very expensive and many of them sought out long-term treatment, surgeries, and purchased their medications on trips back to Mexico. Half of the women cited travel and transportation issues as a problem for them seeking health care, and lastly 2 out of the 10 noted they were "fearful of government action" or deportation out of the U.S.A. if they identified themselves as illegal aliens under American law.

In our research's random interview sampling, the group of 14 Zimbabwean women had sought out emergency care 16 times more than their 10 Mexican female counterparts, with the interviewed Zimbabwean women totaling an average of 4.8 visits, while surveyed Mexican women averaged 2.3 visits. This was due, at least in part, to the average stay of Mexican women in the United States being 8 times longer than their Zimbabwean counterparts in South Africa, with Mexicans at 6.8 years (or 81.6 months) to the average Zimbabwean woman's stay of 10.7 months. All of the combined undocumented Mexican and Zimbabwean women's reported symptoms, treatment, and identified diagnoses were noted in the one-on-one interviews. Not surprisingly, the two collective groups utilized obstetrical and gynecological care more than any other emergency healthcare service. Since the median ages of both groups, Zimbabwean at 31.1 and Mexican at 33.9, were within child-bearing age, the use of obstetrical care by half of the women was not

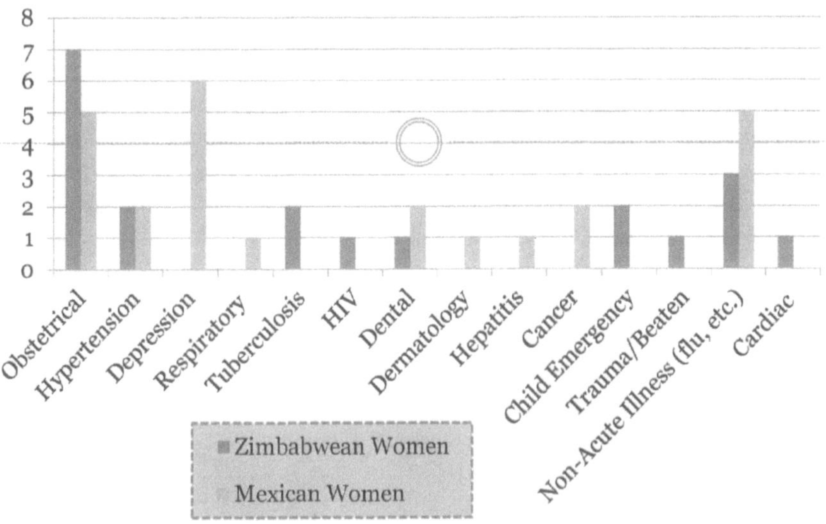

Figure 6.3 Utilized Healthcare Services by Interviewed Zimbabwean and Mexican Women in Host Country

unanticipated. Aside from the ostensible need for obstetrical care among women of child-bearing ages, several women noted seeking gynecological care due to issues such as hemorrhaging, diagnosed but untreated non-malignant fibroid tumors, pelvic pain, and menorrhagia (menstrual periods where bleeding is abnormally heavy or prolonged) (see Figure 6.3).

When we divided out the emergency services sought by the two groups of Mexican and Zimbabwean women, some interesting variations were noted. The type of emergency health care that was sought out by both of these groups of women proved somewhat analogous in the arenas of obstetrical care, dental, hypertension (high blood pressure), and non-acute illnesses (like the basic flu, migraine, manageable diarrhea, etc.). For instance, the two reported cases of hypertension were equivalent comprising the two groups of Mexican and Zimbabwean women. Only the interviewed Zimbabwean reported seeking care for cardiac (high acuity) issues, trauma from being robbed or beaten, and the high acuity, and infectious diseases of HIV/AIDS and tuberculosis. Due to the social stigma of reporting HIV/AIDS and the total voluntary nature of the interviews, there can be extremely minor rates of transparency expected in the self-reporting of such illnesses and diseases.

Another significant difference among the Mexican and Zimbabwean woman was the Mexican women's use of an American Emergency Room for the treatment of a low-acuity illness. Half of the interviewed Mexicans sought care for lower-acuity illnesses such as diarrhea, flu, and migraines compared to less than one-quarter of the Zimbabweans. For instance, undocumented Mexican women sought out care for lower acuity dental emergencies at twice the rate of the interviewed Zimbabwean women. Of note was the decidedly consequential variation in the cited illness' acuity and communicability/infectious nature. For the purposes of this research, an infectious (or high-acuity) disease will be classified as a disease caused by a microorganism or other agent (such as a bacterium, fungus, or virus) that has acute, chronic, and/or potentially life-threatening symptoms or outcomes. While it would prove scientifically unviable and irresoluble to place each woman's disease and/or illness precisely within the confines of only two groupings of 'acute' (high severity) versus 'non-acute' (low severity) illnesses—an attempt was made to note the various illnesses as either infectious (more evident as acute by the tangible disease's classification) or non-infectious, non-chronic, and non-acute by nature. For the purposes of this research, we will define a chronic illness as a condition that usually lasts 12 months or longer and places limitations on self-care and independent living, and/or causes the need for ongoing treatment with medical products, services, and/or specialized medical equipment. While some groupings may have proven more problematic, some were relatively discernible by their easily distinguishable nature. Some low-acuity classifications included back pain, headache (migraine), urinary tract infection, sinusitis/bronchitis/upper respiratory infection (URI), minor laceration, dental pain, an abscess, or rash, etc. More communicable (and high-acuity) diseases (such as Tuberculosis and HIV/AIDS) were cited by the interviewed Zimbabweans than the interviewed Latinas.

For instance, to classify the flu as 'low acuity,' even though its' modality may well fall within the confines of a 'contagious' classification, it is evident as it falls outside of the parameters of a (typically) severe, chronic, or life-threatening illness to a normal, healthy person without any pre-existing chronic healthcare issues (such as asthma, TB, HIV/AIDS, etc.). The lower-acuity level patient is usually not admitted to the hospital, will not receive advanced imaging studies (like CT scans or MRIs), and no complex work-ups with blood tests, etc. They may receive one or two simple ancillary tests (like X-ray or a single lab test), but no more. Conversely, high-acuity patients are usually admitted to the hospital or some long-term care facility, receive advanced imaging studies (like CT scans or MRIs), and (more) complex work-ups with blood tests, etc. Therefore lower acuity patients, more times than not, could easily have been treated at a lower-level clinic (Americans have dubbed these stand-alone 24-hour emergency clinics as a "doc-in-the-box"), where such appropriate care environments are accessible and affordable. Unfortunately, these so-called 'doc-in-a-box' American stand-alone 24-hour emergency clinics will (generally speaking) only treat insured patients, or uninsured patients who have life-threatening emergencies and must be treated immediately. This research should not be misconstrued as a commentary as to whether or not these patients *should* be in an ED. In America's current healthcare environment, they are oftentimes forced to seek out care in the ER as they have no other healthcare facility available to them. The ED personnel have a sacrosanct duty as the 'care provider of last resort'—always available, no matter what. Nonetheless, the use of any high-level ED at a major public or private hospital for primary-level clinical care is a terribly expensive, uneconomical, and superfluous waste of resources. In comparison to a primary care clinic, the fixed costs of staffing, equipping, and operating a high-level trauma center equipped with advanced imaging, and an Intensive Care Unit, are apparent. From a fiscal and public healthcare perspective, the distinction between higher-cost, long-term, chronic, and infectious diseases versus minor illnesses that congest an ED cannot be disregarded.

Complexities in Hormones and Pain

Generalizations can also be made that women's physiology comprises greater biological complexity than men, in that women experience more lifelong fluctuations in hormones due to the menstrual cycle, pregnancy, and menopause, and also undergo more alterations in body weight during their lifecycle than men. These fluctuations have been shown to lead to a compromised immune system, which can manifest symptoms relative to diseases and illnesses, hence the greater use of medical services among females. It has also been observed that intense stress weakens a person's immunity and that women are much more susceptible to autoimmune disease than men (Mark 2005). Mark also notes that these gender differences reduce with age, but persist until at least age 65.

There are some complexities that female hormones add to the emergency medicine and treatment of trauma and disease, namely pain and pregnancy. Pain perception in women has been shown to fluctuate depending on their hormonal state. During the latter stages of pregnancy, women have been shown to have higher pain thresholds than at other times. Also pain thresholds are lower during the luteal, or latter, phase of the menstrual cycle when compared to the follicular (or proliferative) phase, during which follicles in the ovary mature—although overall women show more pain sensitivity than men (Wiesenfeld-Hallin 2005). Some psychosocial factors specific to women have been identified that may also increase their sensitivity to pain, including hypervigilance (increased perception of threats), greater body monitoring, and increased incidence of anxiety and depression. These hormonal issues are necessary for EMS and response crews to keep in mind so that pain acuity, patient presentation, and treatment can be assessed and administered more effectively to women.

Complications in Pregnancy

The pregnant state adds its own set of variables to this biological-makeup mix. For instance during pregnancy, gastric emptying and gastric acid production are reduced, the plasma volume increases by 50%, total body water increases by 7–8 liters, body fat increases 20–40%, renal function and clearance rise, increasing the elimination of many drugs (Langley 2003). Depending on the nature, impact, and length of the forced migration or refugee scenario, women can develop high rates of premature births, vaginal infections, and pregnancy losses due to the disruption of public healthcare infrastructures, which are critical for proper prenatal, intrapartum, and postpartum care. Under normal circumstances approximately 15% of pregnant women require emergency obstetrical treatment, but in disasters and refugee emergencies, this number rises significantly. For instance during 2005s Hurricane Katrina it has been estimated that there were over 200,000 evacuees. More than 1.1 million women of reproductive age (15–44 years) resided in the affected areas before the storm, and overall some 56,000 pregnant women and 70,000 infants were directly affected by the storm (Callaghan et al. 2007). Callaghan et al.'s research also noted that disruptions in clean water supplies for drinking and bathing, inadequate access to safe food, interruption of health care, crowded conditions in shelters or refugee camps, and disruption of public health and clinical care infrastructure were all factors that posed threats to these vulnerable populations.

Aside from the obvious need for specialized obstetrical medical care, pregnant and lactating women should be provided supplementary supplies and services, such as private breastfeeding and OB/GYN exam areas, daily prenatal nutritional advocacy, sterile delivery supplies, prenatal vitamins, pregnancy testing supplies, ultrasound and OB/GYN services, and breast-feeding pumps (see the complete Gender-Aware Disaster Care in chapter 7). The critical nature of daily post-disaster prenatal nutritional advocacy was reported in Jamaica after Hurricane Gilbert when post-disaster prenatal maternal diets were shown deficient in folic acid and the incidence of neural tube defect births increased significantly (Buekens 2006). It should also be noted that religious and patriarchal practices may preclude a woman's receipt of life-saving obstetrical and gynecological care due to a lack of female physicians for female OB/GYN care for necessary pelvic exams (Mantilla 2005); therefore, it is imperative that female gynecologists be available in post-disaster areas where these traditions are practiced.

In the high-stress environment of post-disaster shelters and settings, breastfeeding can become an unmanageable and time-consuming challenge. Researchers found that only 7% of infants in Hurricane Katrina-affected states were breastfed the recommended 12 months, compared with 17.8% nationally, so the hurricane affected a large number of pregnant women and infants already at high risk for adverse outcomes (Callaghan et al. 2007). A significant concern lactating women have in post-disaster settings is their exposure to contaminated and dirty flood waters, unsafe foods, and unclean water. The Center for Disease Control and Prevention (CDC) has studied this issue and continues to advocate breastfeeding despite the potential presence of chemical toxins. Their position is that for most women and their babies the benefits of breastfeeding outweigh the risks, though the toxicity of chemicals may be most dangerous during the prenatal period and the initiation of breast-feeding. The CDC notes that the effects on the nursing infant "have been seen only where the mother herself was clinically ill from toxic exposure" (CDC 2007). It should be noted that unknown environmental exposures can take years to assess and manifest themselves in causality and toxicity. One study by Janerich and his associates examined suspected environmental hazards, tracking leukemia, lymphoma, and spontaneous abortions following floods in New York. Their findings concluded that the median interval between a disaster and a confirmed diagnosis was over one year (1981). For now, one must endorse the current CDC recommendations. Nevertheless, this is where our lack of gender-specific disaggregated data is an impediment and a distribution of post-disaster information on breastfeeding and environmental exposures would assist healthcare providers and women to clarify this critical issue.

Aside from environmental exposures to their pregnancies, post-disaster women face physiological and biological exposures due to their physiological (anatomical) makeup, as well as biological processes and pharmacological challenges in menstruation and contraceptive use. Women who have been forced to wade through water contaminated by corpses, chemicals, and sewage are anatomically vulnerable to genital rashes and vaginal infections. If a menstruating woman with an inserted tampon wades through contaminated water, it is possible for toxic substances to be absorbed through the tampon into her vagina, possibly leading to infections, and even toxic shock syndrome (Richter 2008). Globally, about 52% of the female population (26% of the total population) is of reproductive age, with the majority girls and women menstruating two to seven days every month, according to WaterAid.org's report "Menstrual Hygiene Matters: A Resource for Improving Menstrual Hygiene around the World" (2012). But due to the stigma and universal silence that usually accompanies menstruation, solutions for menstrual hygiene management is typically a low priority. The same WaterAid study reported that this 'Cycle of Neglect' impacts women and girls in several ways, including, but not limited to, a lack of involvement in decision-making in water management and emergency relief planning (purchase of feminine hygiene products or use of wash/toilet facilities to wash sanitary materials); lack of social support (taboo to touch water points, or prepare food, religious activities, etc.); lack of information and awareness (no knowledge of biological processes or effective/safe hygiene practices); and a lack of access to feminine hygiene products and toilet/water facilities; and an adverse impact on girls' education (missed days of schooling) (WaterAid 2012). Even today's "modern" twenty-first century women have many taboos and religious restrictions placed on this naturally occurring event. For instance: Russian Orthodox Christians seclude women during menstruation and they are not allowed to attend church services or have contact with men; Coptic Christians in Ethiopia do not permit menstruating women to enter a church or kiss religious icons; in Judaism menstruating women cannot pass an object to a man, share his bed, eat from the same plate. There are also countless tribal or local taboos, curses and "evil spirits" that surround menstruation. Just a few examples from WaterAid.org's report include: In Tanzania, some believe that if a menstrual cloth is seen by another, the owner can be cursed; in Bangladesh, women bury their cloths to prevent them being used by "evil spirits"; in Sierra Leone, it is believed that used sanitary napkins can make you (or another) sterile; in Surinam, menstrual blood is "dangerous" and you can do harm to a menstruating woman by using black magic, and so on. It is these socio-cultural factors that further restrict forced migrant and post-disaster women to safely manage their menstrual hygiene without access to medical help. Medical assistance can be needed for: severe pain during periods (Dysmenorrhea); excessive, very heavy, and prolonged bleeding (also known as Menorrhagia) which can lead to anemia and be fatal if left untreated; too-frequent menstruation (Polymenorrhea); a lack of menstruation (Amenorrhea); very light menstruation (Oligomenorrhea); and/or spotting (inter-menstrual bleeding)—symptoms which can conceal serious and even life-threatening issues like fibroid tumors, malignant tumors, cervical or uterine cancer, and more. Poor menstrual hygiene (the re-use of unclean products, improper materials, etc.) can allow bacteria to cause local infections and/or travel up the vagina and enter the uterine cavity—which can lead to toxic shock syndrome, pelvic inflammatory disease, bacterial vaginosis, urinary tract infections, yeast infections such as thrush (candidiasis), and other acute illnesses. It is these cultural practices, taboos, and emergency management sanitation issues around menstruation that continue to adversely impact women's health, reinforce and bolster gender inequities, and increase a woman's social exclusion.

In an effort to more effectively meet the needs of women, disaster planners and responders must plan for the provision of a range of feminine antifungal and hygiene products (varieties of types and sizes of sanitary pads and tampons), as well as a selection of new undergarments. Information on vaginal infections, toxic shock, and environmental contamination could be addressed through the distribution of 'fact sheet' to female evacuees of menstruation age. Time and again in disaster response, we have witnessed post-disaster vaginal infections and many women who suffer in silence due to perceived or real social stigmatization, a lack of knowledge concerning gynecological issues, and insufficient or non-existent menstrual, antifungal, and feminine supplies.

Now that we have reviewed some of the primary concerns in women's health and disease, let us examine some psychosocial and mental health differences between men and women and their impacts in post-disaster scenarios.

MENTAL HEALTH AND GENDER-BASED VIOLENCE

Although oftentimes overlooked, emergency room visits and emergency mental health conditions—either due to physical symptoms (like heart palpitations or elevated blood pressure) or a mental condition—can constitute a significant portion of female forced migrants' ER and EMS patients. Factors to consider in assessing the mental health of forced migrants include: the patient's attitude to illness; migration status, experience, phase, and adjustment; the host society's attitudes; cultural identity and conflict; ethnic density; and achievements and expectations (Bhugra and Jones 2001). Cultural challenges can include, but are not limited to, ethnic and/or tribal differences and historic friction, religious prohibitions, acculturation, a patient's "health literacy" (their general knowledge or awareness of physiological and mental health subject matter), pre-existing ethnic relationships, and more.

Psychosocial differences between men and women and their impacts in post-disaster/post-migration scenarios can vary widely, dependent upon each individual and their experiences. Symptoms of PTSD may be difficult initially to distinguish from normal grief reactions, but are manifest by long-term effects (over 30 days) from the event. Sometimes these symptoms last for years, sometimes they last for a lifetime. They include persistent hyperarousal, avoidance, confusion, and/or re-experiencing the event. These effects can lead to extreme anxiety reactions and real physical "emergency" symptoms such as hyperventilation, shortness of breath, headaches, chest constriction, as well as elevated blood pressure, and heart rate. PTSD from disasters can lead to profound long-term effects, affecting a person's immunity, health, and quality of life. Components of a Mexican or Zimbabwean female refugee that are more likely to cause PTSD include any situation that evoked feelings of intense fear, helplessness, and/or hopelessness such as a near-death experience, witnessing a traumatic death or severe injury, rape and/or assault.

Due to the extreme violence witnessed by Mexican and Zimbabwean women, severe stress, PTSD, and mental trauma can be expected. The National Association for the Care of the Handicapped in Zimbabwe stated that violence will continue to haunt its victims, and society, long after the violence ends: "Limbs have been severed and mutilated, thus adding to the physical disability population. People have been subjected to such brutal head injuries that their sight and hearing has been affected, while some have been traumatized so much by the intensity and brutality of the violence that they have joined the ranks of the mentally challenged" (NASCOH 2008).

There are numerous reported differentiations in PTSD's manifestations, risk factors and rates between men and women. PTSD rates among women have been reported up to twice as often as rates among men, with profound differences in its manifestations (Yehuda 2001). At patient presentation (ER or EMS patient assessment), men tend to show more aggression and impulsive behaviors and have more substance abuse issues, while women often present with symptoms of numbing and avoidance and manifest more mood and anxiety issues. Most men experience PTSD after physical violence or on-the-job trauma, whereas women are more likely to have a history of rape or physical assault. Other lifelong risk factors that seem to make women more vulnerable to PTSD include past unwanted sexual contact, the responsibility of being the primary caretaker in the household, concerns for the community at large, and a history of recent mental and emotional issues (Pulcino et al. 2003). Some researchers have reported there are "marker" symptoms often apparent early on that may preclude full-blown PTSD, include re-experiencing the traumatic event and hyper-arousal manifested as peri-event panic (Stuber et al. 2006). Stuber defines peri-event panic as "sudden and unexpected discrete periods of intense fear or discomfort in the hours after a traumatic event" (2006, 55), and that early interventions targeting women with marker symptoms might mitigate the progression to full-blown PTSD.

Notwithstanding PTSD and other mental disorders, perhaps one of the most interesting findings of this research was the rather high number of the interviewed Mexican (6 out of 10) women citing depression as their indication for seeking emergency health care. We should comprehensively examine the extreme variances in the reported variances of this particular illness. Latinos, or Hispanics, are currently the largest minority group in the United States, and Mexican-Americans form the largest subgroup with approximately 6 in 10 Latinos. These Hispanics, according to 2005 study, face disparities in the recognition and treatment of major depression, and the under-recognition of depression in adult Hispanic Americans may be related to language differences, health literacy barriers, somatic presentations, and use of cultural idioms of distress, according to Lewis-Fernández et al. (2005). 'Circular' migratory repetition—especially by the frequent back-and-forth travel of Houston-based Mexicans to Mexico—helps maintain Mexican migrants' touchstone of their culture of origin. Latinos are twice as likely to seek help for mental health problems from primary care providers (which is oftentimes their emergency room physician), than from mental health specialists, as their use of these specialists is significantly lower than that of majority whites (Lewis-Fernández et al. 2005). The study also noted that the Hispanic's expression and presentation of symptoms to an American healthcare provider can be based on cultural articulations and jargon-based ethnic terms:

> Many depressed Hispanics present to primary care and specialty mental health complaining of other culturally patterned idioms of distress. These are linguistic and bodily styles of expressing and experiencing illness, and affliction more generally that do not have a one-to-one relationship with diagnostic categories. Many low-income Hispanics, for example, describe a constellation of depressive, anxiety, somatic, and dissociative symptoms known as *nervios* (nerves) illness. With some gender, age, and Latino subgroup variation, reports of *nervios*

> typically signal particular patient and family expectations about causation, symptoms (eg, trembling, fatigue, malaise, "brain-ache" (*dolor de cerebro*), perceptual distortions such as hearing noises or seeing shadows (known as *celajes*), treatment, outcome. Knowledge of these cultural idioms can facilitate rapport and psychoeducation, help justify and guide the diagnostic work-up and minimize the risk of misdiagnosis. (Lewis-Fernández et al. 2005, 289–90)

This research's unexpected finding on depression begs the question: Why is the forced migrant experience with depression between the interviewed Mexican and Zimbabwean so disparate? Six out of 10 of the interviewed Mexicans reported depression, but not a single interviewed Zimbabwean woman did. Perchance the results have been skewed and obscured through social stigma, communication snags, cultural idioms, or a lack of mental health literacy? This research's results run contrary to Zimbabwe's suggested high rates of depression, so further investigation into this finding was warranted. According to the Zimbabwean Ministry of Health and Child Welfare (2013), depression is among the top five mental health illnesses seen in public health institutions. And from many accounts and reports, the rates of depression among Zimbabweans, either in-country or in South Africa, are substantial, and on the rise.

The United Nation's Integrated Regional Information Networks (IRIN) News (a humanitarian news and analysis service from the UN Office for the Coordination of Humanitarian Affairs) reported in September 2007, that approximately 40% of Zimbabwe's 12 million people, or more than a third of the country's population, were suffering from poor mental health, according to Dr. Dickson Chibanda, a psychiatrist formerly employed by Zimbabwe's health ministry. Chibanda attributed the high level of psychomatic ailments to the country's seven-year long economic crisis, fear of being arrested, living under extreme poverty, unemployment, experiencing hunger, living far from home and families, and Operation *Murambatsvina* (Clear Out Trash—a slum clearance by ZANU-PF in 2005 in which homes and markets were demolished, leaving more than 700,000 people reportedly homeless). The same report noted a significant increase in Zimbabweans consulting traditional healers for mental health problems: "Our records show that traditional medicine practitioners are being visited every day by people who display clear signs of mental disorders; there is a definite rise in people affected," stated Gordon Chavunduka, president of the Zimbabwe National Traditional Healers Association (IRIN 2007). Furthermore, Chavunduka noted that there is a "general belief that mental problems are caused by evil spirits, most of our patients, the majority of whom come from poor backgrounds, say they have severe stress and depression owing to problems caused by economic hardships." It is apparent that stressors such as family breakdowns (spouses had moved to other countries seeking employment), or household disputes due to unstable living conditions, would increase anxiety, depression, and distress. We differentiate stress as two categories: eustress (a "good" stress that can motivate and invigorate) and distress (when stress becomes intolerable, unbearable, and unmanageable to the person). Distress can precede poor decision making, usher in physiological symptoms like in high blood pressure, rapid breathing, and tension, and lead to changes in behavior like overeating, loss of appetite, drinking, smoking, and other adverse coping mechanisms (drug use, etc.), according to Brock University (2013).

As for gender variations, the University of Zimbabwe Medical School in Harare study noted higher rates of depression among Zimbabwean women. This report, published by the University of Zimbabwe Medical School as "Depression in Developing Countries: Lessons from Zimbabwe," noted that depression, as a form of mental illness, was common in an environment of "absolute poverty" and substandard public health services (2001, 482). The researchers in the same study noted that amongst the adult population seeking primary medical care, one-quarter of the people at clinics and hospitals, and one-third attending traditional healers, had depression, and women were "more affected" than men, with women's anxiety disorders at 15.7%, and rates of postnatal depression at 16% (2001, 482). According to the same aforementioned University of Zimbabwe study, somatic complaints (like headaches, malaise, and fatigue) were the most common presentations of depression, but Zimbabwean patients did, after further questioning, acquiesce to having mental and emotional symptoms also:

> Many somatic symptoms, especially those related to the heart and the head, are cultural metaphors for fear or grief. Most depressed individuals attribute their symptoms to "thinking too much" (*kufungisisa*), to a supernatural cause, and to social stressors. Our data confirm the view that although depression in developing countries often presents with somatic symptoms, most patients do not attribute their symptoms to a somatic illness and cannot be said to have "pure" somatisation. This means that it is vital to understand the culture specific terminology used by patients. (University of Zimbabwe Medical School 2001, 483)

The University of Zimbabwe Medical School's report also noted that in Zimbabwe the word "depression" is used almost exclusively to signify an physical illness, which rarely would present itself as an emotional symptom(s). Therefore, there is an incongruity concerning the term and its applicability for healthcare workers and their patients. The same research stated that "case records that require health workers to state a diagnosis show far lower numbers of depression than is expected from epidemiological studies" (2001, 482). This observation would, indeed, explain the non-existent numbers of reported cases of depression among the 14 interviewed Zimbabwean women. While conducting the interviews, even with a Shona interpreter, there may well have been a terminology miscommunication and cultural misinterpretation due to an American medical healthcare worker asking a Zimbabwean woman about "feeling sad" or being "depressed."

Considering the culture-specific concepts of mental illness, the training of international or non-native health workers should include the identification and incorporation of these concepts in conjunction with the overall medical evaluation. A patient's lack of health literacy, as well as general mental and physiological health knowledge are all significant challenges to overcome as healthcare providers. In conclusion, it is this research's finding that the vast disparity of reported depression between the interviewed Mexican and Zimbabwean women was due, by and large, to three or more factors: an incongruous communication clash of a Western biomedical model of depression and the Zimbabwean cultural concepts of depression as a medical disorder; high domestic violence reporting among the Mexican women; a general lack of mental health 'literacy' and how mental health disorders interact with physiological symptoms and behavioral mechanisms among Zimbabwean women; and conceivably a low recognition or consequence for mental health problems in contrast to the Zimbabwean woman's grave day-to-day survival challenges.

In post-disaster and forced migration settings, where chaos rules and there is a breakdown of normal social authority, women can find themselves vulnerable to a variety of physical and sexual threats that can cause PTSD, including rape. According to Fothergill, accounts of sexual and physical assaults should be viewed within the framework of the "gendered nature" of disasters, forced migration, and risk exposures that some women experience as a result of gender inequality, lack of resources, lack of mobility, and a loss of social support structures (1996). The loss or interruption of normal healthcare (clinic or hospital) and emergency (police, fire, EMS, etc.) services makes the prevention, treatment, and reporting of these crimes more difficult. In other words, in the chaos and social breakdown that accompanies refugee migration and disasters, "women become uniquely vulnerable to sexual abuse, including rape and gang rape" (Chew and Ramadas 2005, 2). There are many causes that can contribute to sexual violence, and several that have been reported by the UNHCR include male perpetrators power and domination over their female victims; psychological stress of refugee life; absence of communal support systems; crowded facilities or shelters; lack of physical protection; general lawlessness in facilities and shelters; alcohol and drug use; politically motivated violence against displaced persons; and single female separated from male family members (1995).

In disaster scenarios, where chaos rules and there is a breakdown of normal social authority, rape can occur. For any variety of reasons women in post-disaster settings may feel or become unable to carry on their pregnancies, so family planning support is imperative. Family planning can be an important part of disaster planning, and according to the World Health Organization, over 123 million women from around the world have expressed a desire to control, space, or limit their births (Campbell 2005). In order to meet this need different types of contraceptives (including 'morning-after' pills, condoms, and oral contraception choices), pregnancy testing kits, rape kits, on-site (or readily accessible) sexual/domestic violence counselors, and sexually transmitted infection (STI) testing and treatment should be made available.

The physical care and psychological treatment of women is especially critical in cases of rape. South Africa has one of the highest incidences of rape, with 76 per 100,000 women reporting rape in 2007, compared to 30 women per 100,000 in the U.S.A. (Fuller 2010). Mbuyiselo Botha, from the South African Men's Forum, which campaigns for women's rights, told the BBC's Focus on Africa programme, "It means that we continue in South Africa to be one of the highest capitals of rape in the world. I don't think it's cultural per se; I think it has to do with how a lot of us men worldwide were raised. The issues of dominance against women, issues of inequality, are pervasive and you find them throughout the world" (BBC 2009, 1). In an interesting pro-active twist, a native South African woman, Sonnet Ehlers, created the Rape-a*X*e system, an anti-rape device that consists of a latex sheath with razor-sharp barbs. The anti-rape device is worn like a tampon and when an attacker attempts vaginal penetration the barbs attach themselves to the penis. The device must be surgically removed, which results in the identification and arrest of the attacker. The controversial device has both its supporters and detractors, with some arguing that the device is inhumane, could potentially further enrage the rapist, and cause (more) physical violence to the rape victim.

In conclusion, how all of these complexities in gender-based biology may be applied and implemented into more effective and pro-active female refugee care and post-disaster settings have yet to be conclusively researched and determined. But clearly time is of the essence in establishing gender-based healthcare policies, particularly in light of the serious threefold threat of refugee and natural disasters, and pandemics (such as the swine and avian bird flu, and HIV/AIDS). As we've seen, current research points to increasing exposures and losses in disasters, with impacts becoming demonstrably more pronounced due to ongoing social, political, and economic issues that dramatically and adversely affect women's health care. When we fail to effectively address gender-based healthcare policies, we trigger a potential environment rife with unnecessary suffering, disabilities, and slower recoveries for female forced migrants and disaster victims. As we conclude our look at health and disease among female Zimbabwean and Mexican undocumented refugees and migrants, we see that women do suffer from many of the same diseases and illnesses as men, but they endure them uniquely as women. Today's gender-based disaster research should not only seek to identify issues, but emphasize feasible interventions which could significantly reduce pain, suffering, and long-term post-disaster care costs. Gender-based disaster awareness combined with the application of effective supplies, services, and interventions will allow planners and providers to take a more cognizant and proactive approach to gender-specific needs assessment, care, and advocacy. As an emergency care provider, my coworkers and I have a duty to assist all patients, and this includes a fight against the marginalization of women in refugee emergency healthcare planning and provision programs. Indeed today it is no longer a question of whether women have gender-distinctive healthcare concerns and needs during and after disasters, and in relief efforts—it's a question how we can research, recognize, and react to these differences, and impart equity, access, and more effective treatment for undocumented women in emergency health care.

Chapter 7

A Chance for Change

This chapter will provide an overview of selected pioneering policies that have accomplished positive transformation(s), and explore progressive changes that can take place in gender/social relations following a disaster or forced migration, including innovations to alleviate ED overcrowding. New gender-friendly healthcare politics and forced migration policies by various human rights organizations will be addressed, seeking to find core legal and practical arguments that could enable legal entry, regularization of status and temporary work status, and the possibility of no further forced deportations.

As we have reviewed previously, sudden-onset natural disasters can be viewed as an unprejudiced "leveler," in that they strike as nondiscriminatory weather-based forces—but post-disaster populations are affected disproportionately—in that poor infrastructures are decimated, infrastructures primarily populated by the poor and politically marginalized. Notably, "entirely man-made disasters, such as wars, display even greater spatial and political bias" (Gunewardena and Schuller 2008, p. ix). According to Nandini Gunewardena and Mark Schuller's book, *Capitalizing on Catastrophe: Neoliberal Strategies in Disaster Reconstruction*, post-disaster reconstruction brings into play varying interfaces between nongovernmental humanitarians, for-profit commercial businesses, the real and assumed "benevolence" and capability of a state, and sometimes even, political threats to governments:

> Whenever a community is 'reconstructed' after a disaster, it is a chance for a bureaucracy to register people and bring them more closely into their embrace. A town rebuilt after an earthquake or flood is typically more ordered and sanitary than its predecessor and its residents more enumerated. The control of infectious disease has been a major battleground between citizen and state,

> with governments seeking to exercise coercive powers to control not only the pathogens but their human vectors, and individuals and activists organizations struggling to ensure that health policy does not contradict basic human rights. (Gunewardena and Schuller 2008, p. x)

Furthermore, people continue to question the sensitivity of state institutions to the needs of people who suffer from disasters and whether or not the "assumed" benevolent state (at least as a social ideal) should, or could be, challenged. Unquestionably since the U.S. government-led humanitarian relief debacle of Hurricane Katrina, the American view of a "benevolent" state has been altered, especially via the social media. Perhaps most notably, one Grammy award-winning and popular American rap artist, Kanye West, publicly stated on a Red Cross nationally televised Hurricane Katrina concert benefit: "George Bush doesn't care about black people" (Democracy Now 2005). These seven words seemed to cast dark pallor over Bush's administration that neither the president nor the U.S. administration could remedy, with many American cars exhibiting bumper stickers that stated: "Bush hates black people." The American Federal Emergency Management Agency (FEMA), President Bush, and city and state government officials (like New Orleans Mayor Ray Nagin) were heavily criticized in post-Katrina news, primarily for their slow response, inability to implement timely evacuations and coordinate efforts with other federal agencies, mismanagement, and a lack of preparation, among other contentions of racial bias and social prejudice.

Gunewardena and Schuller go on to note that the general populace is actively shifting its perception and assessment of what roles the state, NGOs, citizens, and private and commercial sectors should play in post-disaster efforts:

> In the intervening decades, the primacy of formal public institutions in a disaster response has been challenged both by nongovernmental humanitarians and by a resurgent private sector, which in their different ways have eclipsed the principle that citizens qua citizens are entitled to protection, relief and restitution in the event of a disaster. The commercial sector, having challenged the concept of the benevolent state, has further challenged the reality of the capable state. (Gunewardena and Schuller 2008, p. xi)

GENDER TRANSFORMATIONS

As for gender-based changes in relations, many transformations can and do take place following a mass migration or disaster. For instance, women can take on traditional male tasks in refugee and post-disaster settings, which could challenge a society's preconceptions of women's capabilities.

These transformative gaps are envisaged in order to "unsettle and challenge taken-for-granted assumptions concerning problematic issues in everyday life" (Denzin 2014, 73), as well as make progressive feminist alterations in women's undesirable or deleterious gender roles. Yet women are often at their most vulnerable when they are forced to flee, often from predatory male behavior, which usually does not stop even when the women reach their destination. As we have reviewed in the case of Central Methodist Mission church, men continued to prey upon the vulnerable Zimbabwean female refugees, even after they had found temporary housing in what many in society would consider a 'safe zone'—a church.

Other changes that can take place in gender relations following a disaster include demographic profile changes in armed conflict situations (more women than men survive) (InterAction 1998); expectations for marriage and children—for instance, post-genocide Rwanda is considering instituting polygamy due to its current 7:3 female to male ratio (Hammer 2006); changes in labor division (such as the purchase of supplies) (InterAction 1998); and an increased political participation and organization (women can see the benefits of working with other women) (InterAction 1998).

Indeed, as some gender and migration theorists point out, vulnerability can also be viewed as a "marker of credibility" (Palmary 2010)—allowing border agencies, NGOs, and other 'outsiders' to view their native homeland experiences as plausible and 'worthy,' or 'deserving,' if you will, of humanitarian aid, empathy (succor), or any beneficial social/political/fiscal intervention(s). Palmary goes on to note that these constructs of vulnerability are even to a certain degree compulsory to employ in order to "counter the culture of disbelief that is endemic in the North," as the appearance of strength, capability, and resilience "may well cast one's testimony in doubt" (2010, 10). This nebulous notion of which migrant's abysmal experience(s) merit (or are 'deserving') of a government, non-governmental agency, or person(s) intercession strikes at the very heart of aid and refuge allowances and parameters. Consequently (based on my years of fieldwork), my supposition is that these dynamic, subjective, and anecdotal considerations can suffer from ill-defined parameters, and, as such, are (to some extent) condemned as 'perpetually indefinable' standards on a widespread global scale. Therefore this pervasive notion among many governmental relief agencies and organizations to concentrate on women as ill-fated victims (rather than a concentration on women's strengths and opportunities in refugee/forced migration scenarios), continues to be utilized. Post-disaster reconstruction efforts can bring about opportunities to transform prior inequalities, and an auspicious hypothesis is that these post-disaster changes in gender roles can provide women a more equitable share of real community power and a heightened social status. Yet, "the historical record confirm that societies neither defend the spaces women create during struggle nor acknowledge the ingenious ways in which women bear new and additional responsibilities" (Meintjes et al. 2001, 8). Genuinely successful post-disaster gender alterations that survive as long-term transformations may best be developed through a means of an organized force, like a coalition or other (political, civil society, etc.) organizational structure (Meintjes 2001, 76).

While the qualitative interviews in this study did not address women's post-migration roles, it does show the kinds of situations faced by women refugees in relatively hostile host countries. In this respect, the conclusions may open the path for different kinds of questions to be asked by others. It is the gendered nature of women's status that has to some extent meant that women have been vulnerable to predation and even flight in conflict situations or situations where destitution would ensue if they stayed at home. It is this that has given them a victim status. However, despite their vulnerability, women have agency and their very flight from home shows this. It requires personal sacrifice and an inner strength that in itself heralds a process of transformation.

Thus, we will review some selected new pioneering policies that have accomplished positive transformation. How these have been implemented will be the subject of discussion. We will also explore progressive changes that can take place in gender/social relations following a disaster or forced migration event, as well as some truly innovative practices that can alleviate the overcrowding of ED and create more effective tools and successful protocols. New gender-friendly healthcare politics and forced migration policies implemented by various human rights organizations will then be addressed. The objective is to find core legal and practical arguments that could include allowances for legal entry, regularization of status and temporary work status, and the possibility of stopping further forced deportations. I will also present a model for cost-effective 'Gender-Aware Disaster Care.' The outcome of this will be a possible checklist for agencies, states, and NGOs to implement in disaster and/or forced migration planning, taking into consideration different conditions in different contexts.

INNOVATIVE IDEAS

A critical issue facing displaced populations and forced migrants—like the Zimbabwean and Mexican women whose experience of emergency health care is the subject of this research—is the patient's lack of a comprehensive medical history and records. This is an especially grave concern among the chronically ill, prescription drug-dependent, acutely drug-allergic and highly complex (multi-organ, multi-disease) medical-care patients. As these women cross borders, they are oftentimes robbed of their possessions—leaving them at a loss to explain to time-pressed EMS or clinic healthcare providers their previous tests and/or diagnoses, efficacious treatment protocols, allergies, drug dosages, etc. While this may, at the outset, seem like a peripheral issue to populations struggling with the day-to-day provision of food, water, and shelter—medical histories of drug and food allergies, and serious pre-existing medical conditions can mean the difference between life and death in an emergency healthcare situation. Regrettably, medical histories and drug/treatment records recorded on paper can easily be lost, stolen, ruined by rain and usage and lack up-to-the-minute updates. Likewise, high-tech gadgetry can be an out-of-reach option for many populations in developing areas. One recent high-tech gadget new on the U.S. market is a credit-card sized USB storage device which stores all types of patient medical information. These types of devices are about 2 mm thick, hold two gigabytes (or more) of information and are no larger than the size of a credit card. The device is plugged into a computer's USB port and contains pre-loaded software that has the user upload their emergency contacts, doctors, medical conditions, prescriptions, allergies, medical tests, living will, photo, and medical history. Another gadget is a medical emergency alert bracelet that has a working USB flash drive that can hold 2 gigabytes (or more) of information, emergency contacts, family history, lists of allergies, and even images of MRIs and X-rays, and EKG readings. These devices normally come with pre-loaded, built-in software that opens automatically when the USB connector is plugged into any Windows PC. These devices could be used by complex/chronic/high-acuity forced migrant/disaster patients and IDPs who would seek care in hospitals and clinics with laptops. The devices are usually waterproof and can stand up to minimal damage, dirt/dust, and the everyday rigors of life in a developing country.

Other innovations and solutions include new products and services that attempt to address and help resolve overcrowding in South African and U.S. EDs by undocumented migrants—both in desperate need of more cost-effective and efficient patient flows—which can help decrease patient wait times, and increase physician, patient, and staff satisfaction. Studies show that Emergency Room patient arrivals, while random, are not unpredictable. Several factors that can be predicted, and even somewhat controlled, are the number of open/available inpatient beds, elective surgery schedules, staffing issues (such as nurse shortage/understaffing), staff scheduling (such as on-call medical specialists), ancillary support, etc. Conversely, the American College of Emergency Physicians stated that the best way to solve ED overcrowding is to "move critical patients to appropriate floors faster" (2009) and stop "boarding" patients, which is a term commonly used in the ED for holding ER patients in the ED who have been admitted into the hospital, which forces ED staff to monitor the holding patients, preventing new ER admissions and severely limiting ED staff from attending to new ED arrivals. The ACEP released three high-impact, low-cost solutions for hospitals to decrease patient boarding: move admitted patients into inpatient areas, with each unit taking a small number of patients; coordinate the discharge of patients before 12 noon, as timely departures can significantly improve the flow of patients and increase open inpatient beds; and coordinate the scheduling of elective and surgical cases, as studies show that an uneven influx of elective patients (heaviest early in the week) is a prime factor in exceeding capacity (ACEP 2009).

One state-of-the-art high-tech enterprise to address ED overcrowding is real-time ER wait-time products and online services. In order to combat some of the ED issues of overcrowding and long wait times, people are coming up with innovative ideas to bypass and circumvent traditional ED patient intake systems. Take for instance Atlanta, Georgia, U.S.A.-based InQuickER, which is a for-profit company that allows users to access up-to-date ER wait times online and for $25 per visit, holds a "virtual" place in line for the ER patient. The user then arrives at the hospital at the Web-appointed time and gets to see an ER doctor within 15 minutes, or the entire hospital visit is free and paid for by the participating hospital (T. Kiley interview, August 31, 2009). Tyler Kiley, CEO of InQuickER, said that the idea behind the company was "not so much a play for efficiency, but more so a play for improvements in customer service and revenue" (2009). Kiley also noted that hospitals gain much-needed revenue in that the average (insured) patient ER visit brings in a marginal $300 profit, and the InQuickER system brings in higher-margin insured patients (collect 60 cents on the dollar) versus (walk-in) self-pay patients (collect 2–3 cents on the dollar). Kiley said that one hospital that has used the InQuickER system has seen a 20% drop in self-pay patients, which has doubled their collections. In the overall review of the InQuickER system, on the positive side, the system seems to generate necessary hospital revenue (with the rate of "free" hospital payouts less than 1 in 1,000 patient visits) (Kiley 2009), on the downside, the system does nothing to "cure" ED inefficiencies, it merely allows hospitals to "cherry pick" select higher-margin ER patients—so while there may be financial gains, the system offers no real free or fair access solution to ED overcrowding, considering that the ER patient who already has no financial means nor insurance can ill afford to pay the upfront $25 per visit fee to enroll in the system. Since my interview in 2009, there have been several new companies to follow InQuickER system's footsteps, and many American hospitals now post their (almost real-time) "ER wait time" on billboards, iPhone applications, and web-based programs. These and other technical innovations that can help assuage the congestion of the ER's in both South Africa and the

United States would be a welcome boon to the many undocumented patients that must wait countless hours for critical care at current overcrowded public health institutions.

One herculean American supporter of advertising ER wait times is the United States government itself—since 2012, hospitals have had to report ED 'wait times' to Medicare, who posts that information on Medicare's (U.S. Department of Health and Human Service) Hospital Compare website. This site has information about the quality of care at over 4,000 Medicare-certified hospitals in the U.S.A. According to the site, Hospital Compare offers two primary goals in its services: to help consumers make decisions about where they get their health care and to encourage hospitals to improve the quality of care they provide (medicare.gov 2013). The service, which is free to the public, collects and dispenses "objective" data gathered by the agency from consumers, Medicare enrollment and claims data, Centers for Disease Control and Prevention (CDC), National Healthcare Safety Network (NHSN), Hospital Consumer Assessment of Healthcare Providers and Systems (HCAHPS) survey, and other government, hospital and patient data-collection tools. Users can instantly pull up (either graphically as a chart or as a word document) a comparison of their local hospitals in six primary aspects of healthcare, including (1) timely and effective care (How often and quickly each hospital gives recommended treatments for certain conditions like heart attack, heart failure, pneumonia, children's asthma, and surgical patients); (2) rates of readmissions, complications, and deaths (how each hospital's rates of readmission and death rates compare with the national rate; how likely patients will suffer from complications while in the hospital; and how often patients in the hospital get certain serious conditions that could have been prevented if the hospital followed procedures based on best practices and scientific evidence); (3) how the hospital uses outpatient medical imaging like CT scans and MRIs; (4) a survey of patient experiences (How former patients responded to a national survey about their hospital experience); (5) number of Medicare patients (how many people with Medicare have had certain procedures or have been treated for certain conditions at each hospital); and (6) information about how much Medicare pays each hospital (medicare.gov, 2013).

In the article "Emergency Department Billboard Waiting Times: A Solution to ED Overcrowding or a Deterrent to Patients?" a Baylor College of Medicine emergency physician explains that many providers in the medical community vehemently oppose advertising wait times to the general public. Bailey argues that hospitals which advertise wait times do so "simply to lure patients away from competing hospitals . . . and that there is substantial concern regarding the accuracy of projected wait times and the potential of hospitals to falsely advertise" (2011, 1). She also points to a study of 50,000 patients that reported the accuracy (using a linear regression model) between reported (actual) and predicted and advertised ER wait times. These varied by 29 minutes, or some 27% (2012). The doctor also noted that these advertised wait times make the jobs of the ED employees even more difficult—setting unfeasible and unreasonable expectations on overly anxious patients and already strained-to-the-breaking-point providers—all trying to function in a demanding, minute-by-minute, ever-changing emergency medicine environment.

As for South Africa, Dr. Gavin Mooney (Professor of Health Economics at the University of Sydney and an Honorary Professor at the University of Cape Town) expressed several proposals in an article in *The Star* newspaper in April 2012: "Something is Rotten in SA Hospitals." In his article, he formulated three recommendations. First, to bring "one of the big teaching hospitals . . . up to speed in terms of quality and care and efficient management and management systems to act as a major demonstration project showing just what the public sector is capable of" (2012, 15). This program could then be emulated and replicated across the country. Mooney concurs that, while it would require substantial funding, the funds spent on the planned pilot program would be money well spent. Secondly, Mooney explains that the inefficiency in the private sector is just as great as that found in public, but dissimilar in that the quality is higher, but the cost of care (much like the United States) is far too high. He noted that these rising costs cannot be sustained and need to be controlled. Lastly, Mooney writes that there is a need for the creation of some SA governmental investigatory body to determine "where all that money is going" as it "cannot be justified in health terms" (2012, 15). In his conclusion, the economist notes how the rising inequality of incomes in SA makes the country one of the "most unequal societies on the planet and more unequal than in 1994" (Mooney 2012, 15).

Mooney's statement is corroborated by the June 13, 2012, report: "South Africa—The Most Unequal Income Distribution in the World" by London-based Euromonitor International (Hodgson). The report stated that South Africa has the highest income inequality in the world as measured by the GINI Index developed by Italian economist Corrado Gini (1884–1965). According to the World Bank, the index "measures the extent to which the distribution of income or consumption expenditure among individuals or households within an economy deviates from a perfectly equal distribution, "and that this distribution is found by a Lorenz curve that "plots the cumulative percentages of total income received against the cumulative number of recipients, starting with the poorest individual or household" (2013). So in simpler terms, a GINI index of 0 represents 'perfect equality' (an unmistakable misnomer) and an index of 100 implies 'perfect inequality,' both impossible statistics, so the truth lies somewhere in-between these two contradictory counterparts.

This GINI Index level has remained "relatively unchanged between 1990 and 2011 . . . is one of the biggest challenges facing the country and has a detrimental impact on the country's economic development and business environment" (Hodgson 2012, 1). Using this GINI Index method, South Africa rates anywhere from (depending on the statistics used) 63.1 to 67.8 (or around 0.7), while the United States is anywhere from 37 (using Paris-based Organization for Economic Co-operation and Development [OECD] data) to 46.9 (using U.S. Census Bureau data) or around 0.4, with a five-year 2006–2010 GINI index at 0.467 (Babones 2012). Apparently, the United States' all-time low of 38.6 was set in 1968, and not so surprisingly, the "most equal" countries in the world are the Scandinavian countries of Denmark (19.4), Norway (19.3), and Sweden (18.1) (Babones 2012). To put it in more illustrative terms, the United States may well be a rather equally divided country of 'haves' and 'have-nots'—with income distribution set half-way between laissez-faire capitalism and a socialist Promised Land.

In a global landmark moment for gender equality and women's rights, the United Nations announced in September 2009 that four existing agencies (UNIFEM, the Office of the Special Adviser on Gender Issues, U.N. Division for the Advancement of Women, and the International Research and Training Institute for the Advancement of Women) would be morphed into a new "super agency" for women. After three years of negotiation, the 192-member U.N. General Assembly in its sixty-third session unanimously voted (resolution A/RES/63/311) to create a more politically powerful and financially stable U.N. agency to address gender-related issues.

In July 2010, the United Nations General Assembly formed UN Women—the United Nations' Entity for Gender Equality and the Empowerment of Women. Some of the directives of this new mega-group agency are to support inter-governmental bodies in their formulation of policies, global standards and norms; to help U.N. Member States to implement those standards (providing technical and financial support to those countries that request it), to forge effective partnerships with public society, and to hold the UN system accountable for its own commitments on gender equality, including regular monitoring of system-wide progress (2013). According to UN Women, the agency "works for the elimination of discrimination against women and girls; empowerment of women; and achievement of equality between women and men as partners and beneficiaries of development, human rights, humanitarian action and peace and security" (2013). On June 28, 2013, UN Women reported that 50 governments had expressed their support via monetary funding commitments at a fundraising event at their headquarters in New York. Maintained by voluntary financial contributions from governments, foundations, corporations, organizations, and individuals, UN Women received approximately $218 million in total contributions from governments in 2012, much less than was needed to fulfill its annual operating budget (target) of $300 million (2013). Nonetheless this under-funded super-group continues to struggle against worldwide gender inequalities in occupational segregation, gender wage gaps, education and healthcare access, sexual and domestic violence and discrimination, as well as political, social, and economic power and parity.

Nonetheless, other NGOs and agencies have also taken on the task of addressing gender issues in disasters, some of which include the Gender Disaster Network (www.gdnonline.org) at Northumbria University; the Gender Disaster Resilience Alliance (www.usgdra.org); Girls in Risk Reduction Leadership (GIRRL—via the Southern Africa Society for Disaster Reduction SASDiR); USAID Women in Development; EPI Global (www.epiglobal.org); Huairou Commission (www.huairou.org); Plan International (www.plan-international.org); and Oxfam International (www.oxfam.org). One high-tech online initiative that visually depicts where disaster risk reduction efforts are globally active is the "Women and Girls on the Map: Resilience Action by Women and Girls" (womenandgirlsonthemap.crowdmap.com). This site was created for the International Day for Disaster Reduction on October 13, 2012, and was developed by a global coalition of four NGOs: the Gender and Disaster Network, Huairou Commission, Plan International, and Oxfam International.

Another gender-disaster initiative was a five-part GDRA-EPI Global collaborative webinar series from July 2012 to July 2013. Five GDRA-EPI Global webinars included "Gender and Disaster Overview" (July 11, 2012); "Gender-based Violence" (October 10, 2012); "Disasters and Women's Health and Hygiene" (January 16, 2013); "Gender and Climate Change" (April 10, 2013); and "Gender, Disaster, Policy and Politics" (July 9, 2013). With multilingual speakers from academic institutions, NGOs and agencies like the UNISDR, Plan International, GDN, GDRA, and others, the webinar series registered up to 110 attendees at each webinar from countries in Asia, Africa, Latin America, Australia, New Zealand, and the United States. Recordings of each of the five webinars were made available free to the public at EPI Global's website at www.epiglobal.org.

Yet another field-tested gender-based initiative to spearhead recovery and reconstruction efforts was the Myriam Merlet, Anne Marie Coriolan and Magali Marcelin Feminist International Camp in Haiti. The camp was named after the three Haitian feminist activists killed in the island's 2010 earthquake. Back in January 2010, the strongest quake in more than 200 years (7.0 on the Richter scale) hit Haiti, a nation where women already suffered from deep-seated inequalities and vulnerabilities such as sexual violence and low prosecution of rape, low socio-economic status, enslavement and human trafficking (WHRD IC 2010). Haitian women's high HIV infection rates (pre-disaster 60%) and estimates of 37,000 pregnant women among the earthquake survivors placed them at high risk for medical emergencies and EMS intervention (WHRD IC and UNFPA 2010). The Myriam Merlet, Anne Marie Coriolan and Magali Marcelin Feminist International Camp was formed in Jimani (along the Haiti-Dominican Republic border) and housed a resource distribution area, a health clinic for women and children, and a communications area, but it also scrutinized and demanded legal action regarding any violations of women's human rights during the earthquake and the aftermath (AWID 2010). Camps that offer gender-aware services and supplies like the Myriam Merlet, Anne Marie Coriolan and Magali Marcelin Feminist International Camp will hopefully be the rule—and no longer the exception—in all future post-disaster outreaches.

POLITICS AND POLICY CREATION

The mass movement of Zimbabwean and Mexican migrants clearly exposes the need for immigration reform and a reconsideration of U.S. and South African asylum policies, politics, and procedures. The social and especially the health problems arising from these mass migrations expose the need to adjust the asylum system in order to more effectively deal with twenty-first century asylum seekers.

According to a June 2008 Human Rights Watch report, there are numerous arguments for the creation of a broad-based policy aimed at ending xenophobia, and regularizing asylum and the presence of Zimbabweans in South Africa. "As resentment among the urban poor against foreigners has grown—with Zimbabweans becoming a prime target of the xenophobic violence which has killed dozens, injured hundreds and displaced tens of thousands—this includes impact on South African social harmony, public safety, and the rule of law" (Human Rights Watch 2008, 3). Human Rights Watch espouses the creation of a policy that would include the permission for Zimbabweans legal entry, regularization of status and temporary work status, and an end to their forced deportation. The group points to eight core legal and practical arguments. These eight arguments contend that regularization would do the following: allow South Africa to meet its fundamental international legal obligations; unburden the asylum system of unnecessary claims; protect Zimbabweans against xenophobic attacks and violence during their entry and stay in South Africa; offset the cost of expensive and ineffective deportation practices and wasteful police resources; provide data on hundreds of thousands of currently undocumented Zimbabweans; assist authorities to enforce minimum wages for employees and create a fair and level employment environment in which South Africans could equitably compete for jobs; directly address Zimbabweans human and public services' needs (emergency room medical aid, education, etc.), thereby reducing the burden on social assistance, NGOs and aid programs; and increase familial support of Zimbabwean family members in Zimbabwe (stemming the flow of refugees) (2008).

The continued mass movement of Zimbabwean and Mexican migrants and other populations is also precipitating substantial changes in other aid-based policies, politics, and procedures. One contemporary program is W.A.S.H.—which stands for Water (and) Sanitation & hygiene. The 2012 UN-Water Global Analysis and Assessment of Sanitation and Drinking-Water (GLAAS) study reported on the ongoing implementation of the UN-Water strategy that is shaping our post-2015 sustainable development arena. According to this report: ". . . the 78 million people still unserved are increasingly hard to reach, and the MDG target for sanitation is not on track: there are currently 2.5 billion people with no access to improved sanitation" (WHO 2012 GLAAS Report, 5). The GLAAS 2012 report asserts that it is "essential to accelerate and sustain services that could ultimately save two million lives per year" especially among forced migrant and post-disaster populations (2012, 5). For instance, Plan India's October 2010 national study revealed that 68% of women in India cannot afford sanitary napkins, only 12% of women use sanitary napkins (others resort to used cloths, husks, sand, ash, and other unhygienic alternatives), and 23% of girls have to suspend their studies due to inadequate sanitation infrastructure in their schools (Khan 2013). According to the World Health Organization, India accounts for 27% of the world's cervical cancer deaths—about twice the global average—doctors declaring poor menstrual hygiene as a substantial factor in the disease (Khan 2013).

Correspondingly, a 2012 WaterAid Report entitled: "Menstrual hygiene matters: A resource for improving menstrual hygiene around the world" reported: "Menstrual hygiene has been largely neglected by the water, sanitation and hygiene (WASH) sector and others focusing on sexual and reproductive health, and education" (WaterAid 2012, 22). Yet there is an increasing identification in W.A.S.H. programs that they must facilitate menstrual hygiene management issues with both privacy and propriety, especially when dealing with inadequate and communal sanitation facilities in schools and other public toilet facilities. Social taboos, religious practices, and a lack of private, feminine hygiene-allocated wash facilities can cause girls to forfeit their class attendance during their entire menstruation cycle. "In order to improve the menstrual hygiene situation for girls over the longer term, menstrual hygiene management needs to become integrated into WASH, as well as education policies and strategies," stated the World Health Organization's 2012 GLAAS report (65). To their healthcare detriment, many countries fail to accommodate and promote women's' access to safe sanitation—and in doing so, a forced migrant women's feminine hygiene needs can remain forfeited and forgotten.

So why do disaster planners and providers seem to fall short of addressing the short-term impacts and long-term effects of disasters on a population's overall health prognoses? Moreover, within the three post-disaster time-frame phases of acute (under one month), intermediate (1–12 months), or long-term (after 12 months) phases fall an overflowing myriad of illnesses, physical and mental traumas, and chronic diseases. Studies show that within the acute phase of patient care infirmities, generally about one half are illnesses, one-fourth are injuries (e.g. cuts, abrasions, sprains, fractures) and other complaints involve routine needs like medication refills, wound maintenance, and assistance in managing chronic health problems like diabetes, hypertension, Congestive Heart Failure (CHF), asthma, etc. (Freedy 2007). One Hurricane Katrina post-disaster study from Tulane University showed that people suffer a myriad of long-term effects on their healthcare when a region's infrastructure is devastated by a disaster (Farris 2011). Several years after the hurricane, the study pointed out that the population's overall health was not improving and that the natural 2005 disaster had generated chronic, life-threatening health implications. "To our surprise, we found a three-fold increase in heart attacks after Katrina, four years later," reported Tulane Interventional Cardiologist Dr. Anand Irimpen, the principal investigator on the study (Farris 2011). Dr. Irimpen of the Tulane University Heart and Vascular Institute explained that many factors have detrimentally impacted this region's health, including unmanaged stress, smoking, increased unemployment, alcohol and drug abuse, crowded living quarters, and the interruption or absence of consistent medical treatment and prescribed drugs—plus an increase in pre-packaged, processed fast foods has led to higher cholesterol rates as well.

The lack of functional gender-based policies (that meet the needs of the kind of stress evoked by the disaster) relates to the lack of an appropriate gender-sensitive framework. EMS and disaster planning need to offer women supplies and services that alleviate both the short-term impacts and long-term effects on this population's overall health prognoses. My own 20-point 'Gender-Aware Disaster Care' compilation of provisions, services, and aids attempts to address and reduce impact, acuity, and costs in post-disaster healthcare provisioning. This gender-aware triage and care intervention provides not merely a checklist, but a systematic approach that will enable services and provisions to be appropriately addressed.

THE 20-POINT "GENDER-AWARE DISASTER CARE" CHECKLIST

1. Create high gender visibility and input throughout all stages of refugee and disaster planning, preparedness, communication, management, response, recovery and reconstruction efforts;
2. Establish a Women's "Principal Point of Contact" Resource Area near/next to OB/GYN assessment & treatment area to create a centralized and efficient "go-to" area for networking with other women; the distribution of gender-aware information & services, female supplies and support that are available (childcare, lactation assistance, sexual & domestic abuse, rape intake, etc.) (Figure 7.1).
3. Provide a private, enclosed "stress-free zone" (no intrusive public eyewitnesses, staffing pathways, or passersby allowances) for an OB/GYN assessment and care area;
4. Ensure daily prenatal nutritional advocacy (check-ups) for all pregnant and lactating women. In order to successfully reduce infant and maternal death and disease, disaster planners, responders and providers should make provisions for nutritional advocacy for mother, fetus and infant. Local emergency managers could ensure compliance of daily prenatal nutritional check-ups by EMS personnel or outsource compliance via local NGOs staff and volunteers. Any nutritional information could be distributed verbally or via written materials at the 'principal point of contact' women's care area;

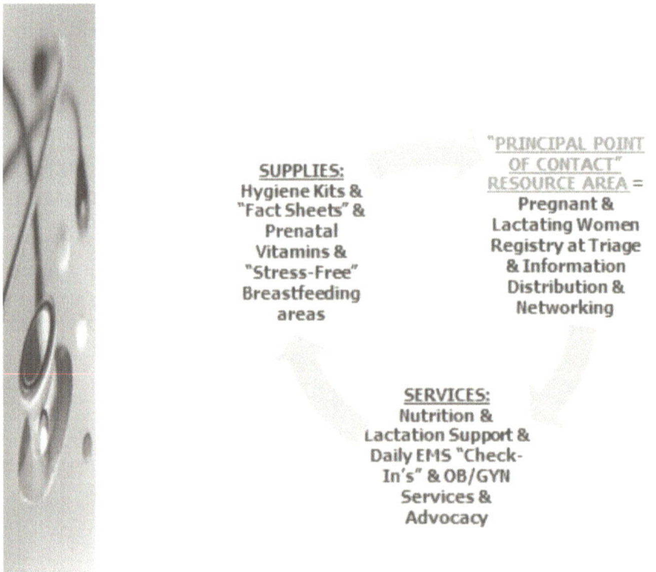

Figure 7.1 Gender-Aware Triage and Care

5. Start a pregnancy registry (at disaster onset—in triage) to track and collect data on any pregnancy complications, miscarriages and birth outcomes. Local emergency managers should ensure compliance of pregnancy registry by EMS personnel;
6. Train non-obstetrical healthcare providers to effectively triage pregnant women. Training could be provided through FEMA, local EMS corps, or NGOs such as Red Cross Disaster Health Services training;
7. Provide a private, tranquil "stress-free zone" (no intrusive public eyewitnesses, staffing pathways, or passersby allowances) breastfeeding area for lactating women;
8. Retain several sterile delivery kits and/or emergency delivery supplies (infant ambu-bag (BVM), blankets, sterile cord clamps and scissors, and other medical requirements);
9. Make provisions for rape intake (rape kits and personnel), as well as onsite (or readily accessible) sexual and domestic violence counselors. Local emergency managers should be responsible for the distribution of information concerning the availability of counseling for these services. Information could be distributed verbally or via written materials at the "principal point of contact" women's care area;
10. Provide prenatal vitamins (folic acid and ferrous sulfate supplements);
11. Provide pregnancy testing supplies, ultrasound and OB/GYN services;
12. Make sexually transmitted disease (STD) testing, information and treatment available. Local emergency managers should be responsible for the distribution of information concerning the availability of counseling for these services. Information could be distributed verbally or via written materials at the "principal point of contact" women's care area;
13. Offer breastfeeding supplies (pumps, pads, etc.) and on-site (or readily available) lactation consultants, as well as ready-to-feed infant formulas;
14. Distribute a 'fact sheet' of information to all pregnant and lactating women on potential effects of vaccines, environmental toxins and exposures on pregnancies and outcomes. Information and these fact sheets could be distributed verbally or via written materials at the 'principal point of contact' women's care area. Some considerations in the presentation of risk information include the audience's understanding of environmental and health risks, language, and possible media or public queries;
15. Distribute a 'fact sheet' to women and girls on all relevant information concerning post-disaster onset, symptoms and treatment of potential vaginal infections, genital rashes, environmental contamination and toxic shock syndrome. Information and these fact sheets could be distributed verbally or via written materials at the 'principal point of contact' women's care area. Emergency managers can further promote dialogue through small group question-and-answer sessions and meetings.
16. Provide a variety of contraception (including 'morning-after' pills, condoms and oral contraception choices) and offer information on any available local family planning on-site or readily available resources;

17. Provide feminine hygiene kits which contain choices of feminine (non-irritating) cleansing wipes, pantie-liners, sanitary pads and/or tampons, as well as bags for discrete storage and disposal. These kits could be distributed at the "principal point of contact" women's care area. In more rural areas and developing nations, these women's and girl's hygiene kits could be produced regionally and from locally resourced and environmentally disposable material;
18. Ensure that female gynecologists and physicians are available in areas where religious/patriarchal/social traditions limit or prohibit non-female physical and/or pelvic exams for women;
19. Have over-the-counter and prescription antifungal yeast infection and genital rash products readily available; and
20. Offer a wide variety (of all sizes) in clean female undergarments.

***

Research supports the contention that many gender-sensitive supplies and services continue to be either inadequate or non-existent in many refugee camps and post-disaster settings. Yet the provision of these relatively inexpensive short-term gender-based interventions could mitigate and even prevent acute illnesses, morbidity, pain and suffering, as well as long-term healthcare costs among female post-migration populations. It can be hypothesized that the stockpiling and provision of these gender-aware supplies and services could serve to decrease the risk for adverse pregnancy and infant outcomes, recurrent healthcare costs and concerns, as well as reducing requirements for multiple medical interventions (ER visits, physician care, etc.). These relatively low-cost, short-term interventions speak to the age-old medical adage, *An ounce of prevention is worth a pound of cure*. Or to coin a new truism, *Take care of them now or see them in the emergency room later*. For instance, without the provision of a private and tranquil breastfeeding area for lactating women, infants can fail to thrive and quickly become dehydrated, so the infant and mother will then be added to the number of patients needing emergency medical attention. Oftentimes it is these early (simple) proactive patient interventions, supplies, and treatments that are averted or disregarded that can prove much more acute (complex) and costly in their latter stages. (See "How Gender-Aware Interventions Can Reduce Impact, Acuity, and Costs," Figure 7.2.)

The Johannesburg-based Consortium for Refugees and Migrations in South Africa (CoRMSA) advocates that greater clarification and investigation be undertaken ensuring the right to health, including ART, of refugees, asylum seekers and other migrants, as outlined in S.A.'s National Department of Health Financial Directive of 2008 (2009). The consortium also seeks a more uniform implementation of the directive across all public institutions

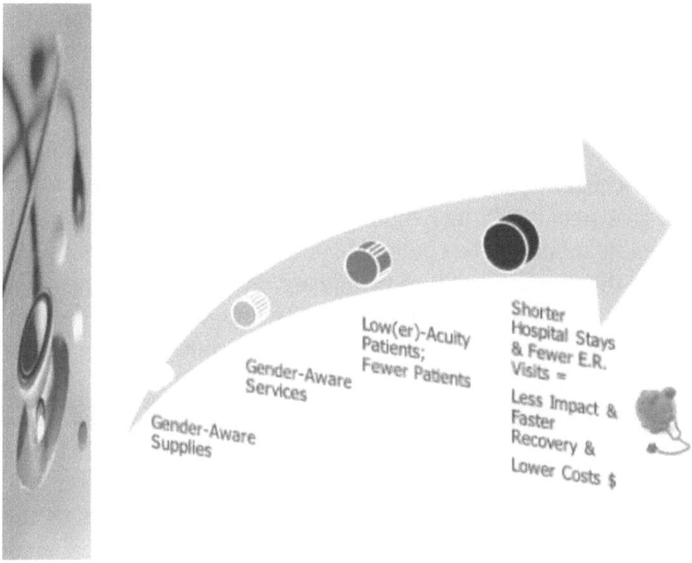

Figure 7.2 How Gender-Aware Interventions Can Reduce Impact, Acuity and Costs

and supports the inclusion of a clause stating that refugees and asylum seekers—with or without a permit—should be exempt from paying for ARV treatment services, irrespective of the of the level of institution (primary or tertiary—including all clinics, community healthcare centers or hospitals).

Some of the experiences of refugees and migrants are a result of a lack of appropriate understanding and therefore of training by healthcare professionals about the needs and rights of their patients. Thus a discernible need exists for compulsory training for all new and existing South African healthcare professionals, nursing school students, and medical university students on xenophobia and healthcare access rights of asylum seekers and refugees. The lack of consciousness for this need means that there is no curriculum among medical training institution to fill this lacuna. There is an urgent need for a curriculum to be created through the National Department of Health and uniformly imposed so that every future medical student and current healthcare provider has a uniform set of instructions via the nation's healthcare system. Perhaps yet another recommendation would initiate the re-certification mandate following the same pattern of BLS, ACLS, ATLS, or CPR training timeframes—so that when and where the healthcare professional's re-certification is mandated, the non-national healthcare rights training would have to be completed in order to become certified or re-certified. A compulsory online course in non-national healthcare rights could also be created and required on a semi-annual, annual, or biennial basis. Special training courses could be administered among healthcare providers in leadership roles, such as hospital administrators, charge/head nurse, chief of staff, and others involved, ensuring the implementation, reinforcement, and compulsory adherence to any and all current refugee and asylum seekers' healthcare rights.

The lack of any widespread awareness campaigns in and among refugee and asylum seeker communities, local churches, refugee camps, schools and NGO affiliates signals a further significant gap. The campaigns could be conveyed in simple terms and be communicated in the refugee's native language, emphasizing the person's right to healthcare, their right to access ART, and could be executed by trusted local community refugee leaders, such as school teachers, associate pastors, women's groups, and other noted neighborhood civic organization leaders. Ideally, these awareness campaigns could be conducted in question-and-answer formats and in small group 'peer-based' supportive settings, rather than larger forums, where privacy, police force, and fear of immigration authority concerns can become an issue.

In conclusion, there are new pioneering policies and programs that have accomplished positive transformations in the arena of gender, emergency healthcare, and forced migration/disaster challenges. In this chapter, we have explored changes that can take place in gender relations following a disaster or forced migration event, looked at some truly innovative high-tech ideas that can alleviate the overcrowding of EDs, and recommended some effective protocols. Fresh legal and practical arguments that included allowances for legal entry, regularization of status and temporary work statuses, and no forced deportations were also addressed. Should states or local authorities implement these processes and programs into their disaster and/or forced migration planning, they could conceivably reduce the impact, acuity and costs to the healthcare system, the aid budgets, and the people.

Chapter 8

A Structural Violation of Human Rights

This final chapter will serve to synopsize how these forced migrant women's suffering is a direct and deplorable consequence of today's current gendered and xenophobic institutionalized public policies, coupled with a failure to enforce healthcare access rights. As activists, medical aid workers and political science researchers, we can draw not only an intangible line—but rather a palpable correlation—between a state's systematic and systemic denial of emergency health care to a structural violation of human rights.

We began this research at the formative cornerstone of 'Ground Zero' in our construction of structural violence, gender equity, ethics of care, human capabilities, GBV, and social composition mechanisms. As explained previously, structural violence was defined as a society or state's potential ability to fulfill an individual's needs, and the structural inequities that result in the lack of fulfillment of those needs. While social inequalities may exist in many communities, events like disasters and forced migration can markedly exacerbate pre-existing social inequities, societal ills, and medical conditions. My preference may be to define structural violence as "macro-proportioned patterns of power" that systemically oppress and exploit individuals—causing unnecessary and continual suffering, disease and death at the "micro-individual" level. Again, it is of significant consequence to differentiate and delineate the pivotal terms *unnecessary, avoidable,* and *continual* when discussing a society or state's potential ability to fulfill an individual's needs and the structural inequities that result in the lack of fulfillment of those needs. As human rights activists and political science theorists, we can draw a dotted line between a state's systematic denials of emergency health care (defined herein as a lifesaving measure) as a structural violation of human rights. Extreme imbalances of social power are based on structural violence (limiting individuals in their quest for equitable access to health care in a society) therefore inequity in the access to lifesaving health care can be regarded as tantamount to structural violence.

This research has attempted to illustrate that not gender—but gender *inequity*—is the mechanism that places girls and women at heightened risks before, during, and after a disaster/ forced migration/refugee crisis. It is acute inequities in social, political, and economic power, cultural roles, and social frameworks that trigger and explode pre-existing structural violence and socially constructed vulnerabilities. A similar and homogeneous declaration can be made on behalf of other vulnerable groups, such as the economically disadvantaged, minorities (and socially marginalized), children, the elderly, the homeless, the disabled, overburdened caregivers, the mentally ill, those with chronic health issues, and so on. At its worst, gender equity pigeonholes women as helpless and hapless victims, tossed about by the caprice of uncompassionate governments and evil men. Gender equity should never seek to become a divisive zero-sum game, in which every word written on female suffering leads to one less word written on male suffering, or vice versa. And certainly gender equity should never seek to condone nor suggest that men remain unaffected by disasters, emergency healthcare issues, and emergencies, instead it should serve as a filtered 'gender lens' that illustrates how men and women are constrained by their socialization and disproportionately impacted by disasters.

At its best, gender equity should seek to highlight and uncover sex- and gender-based differences that might be more effectively harnessed and positively exploited in disaster planning, mitigation, response, emergency healthcare services, and recovery efforts, where women take on roles as capable citizens with gender-specific aptitudes, skilled community competencies, and leadership abilities. Gender equity, accordingly, aims for women's capacity and freedom to (equitably and legitimately) reach their own personal and functional capabilities. This pragmatic approach translates into freedom from oppression, and an enforced (not merely theoretical, but employed and enforced) zero tolerance policy for any political, social, fiscal, or religious subversion or limitations placed on those conferred freedoms.

CULTURES OF CULTIVATION OR ERADICATION?

This research has examined how the application of social justice shapes the demonstrable foundation of public health care—and how it is wholly within the realm of each country's policy makers and healthcare institution's direct and indirect policies and procedures (i.e. culture) to resolve either to passively cultivate or actively eradicate the structural violence of gendered and/or institutionalized xenophobia. Our initial research took an overarching national view of the core concepts, functions, primary goals, and evaluations that establish the parameters for these two host countries' healthcare systems. We then began our review of national public and private healthcare systems in South Africa and the U.S.A., noting the similar and dissimilar core systemic concepts, functions, and goals. Within the comprehensive realm of public health care is emergency health care, and accordingly, a vast majority of healthcare professionals are legally and ethically bound by their public oaths of service to provide lifesaving treatment. Lifesaving healthcare services and treatment (when viable) is often regarded as a fundamental human right, regardless of whether the individual has a means to pay for treatment. This remains a core universal component and principle conviction within the practice of acute/emergency, or lifesaving, health care.

In its most fundamental form, the three core primary goals for health systems, according to the World Health Organization, are set forth as good health, responsiveness to the expectation of the population, and fair financial contribution . . . and that health systems cannot solely be engaged in actions to improve people's health, but also to affect measures that protect populations against the financial costs of illness/disease (2000). The WHO's right to health mandate contains the four so-called AAAQ elements, which include availability, accessibility (non-discrimination and physical, economical and informational accessibility), acceptability (medical ethics and cultural- and gender-sensitive), and quality. Health systems can promote or violate human rights to health care in their design and implementation and vulnerabilities to poor health can be reduced by following the WHO's steps to respect, protect and fulfill people's rights to healthcare systems. Going a step further, Duckett (2004) proposed a simplified two-dimensional approach in how to begin to evaluate healthcare systems: quality, efficiency, and acceptability on one dimension, and equity on another. Undoubtedly investigations that uncover, evaluate, and prevent inequities in healthcare systems remain as critical benchmarks in a nation's system surveillance. Nevertheless inequities in healthcare systems and services continue to exist, disguising themselves as poor physical, economical, or informational accessibility, inequitable treatment, discrimination, or inadequate or disrespectful provider response and treatment. Hence the research indicated that all healthcare providers should unswervingly observe prescribed acuity levels in triage and that these acuity parameters are precise, clinically accurate, and medically relevant—and if uniformly enforced—able to ensure equitable treatment for both the documented and undocumented patient. It is within these decisive life-and-death margins that emergency healthcare decisions for undocumented patient care are being made; therefore it is within these gatekeeper mechanisms that unrecognized patients' emergency health care should commence.

While America currently struggles to put into play its first-ever available universal healthcare system, it continues to offer no explicit constitutional right to health care, and allows each public hospital to struggle with the uneasy ethical decisions of demanding immigration documents (and deny care to any patient who cannot produce them), or to provide unrestricted public healthcare access to any patient in need of care. As the most expensive in the world, the U.S. healthcare system must rein in its excessively high expenditures so that its modern medical technologies, prescription drugs, growth of for-profit hospitals, aging population, uninsured patients, and astronomical administrative costs continue to survive within its hugely complex, multi-tiered payer system. In comparison, South African health care is acutely divided along public and private sector lines—the gaping chasm incontestable to any keen observer's eye. Readily available is an extremely high standard of care in public sector hospitals, replete with state-of-art equipment and training, comparable to and/or exceeding European and American facilities and/or healthcare standards. Nonetheless it is easy to assume how better compensation and working conditions in private hospitals pilfers high-quality doctors and nurses away from the public sector where they are most needed. The South African Constitution guarantees access to health care and other essential services to refugees, asylum-seekers, citizens and migrants, all regardless of legal status. However, in practice, fears of arrest, deportation, and xenophobia, plus a deplorable lack of healthcare literacy, access, and awareness, continues to keep many Zimbabweans from properly gaining usage to these services.

How each nation envisions its own equity and justice in public health care reflects the society's tolerance of inequalities of power. In compelling detail, this research has illustrated that the more financially, socially, and gender-equitable a society is, the more likely its healthcare system will demonstrate equity. And while the provision of public/universal health care remains a significant national challenge for both the United States and South Africa, the health care of refugee and forced migration populations unseals a veritable Pandora's Box of conflicting political, social, fiscal, gender, and human justice issues that politicians, governments, and healthcare providers must grapple with in order to bring its quarrelling viscera under control. As two of the world's top asylum destinations, the United States and South Africa have both teetered between epochs as refuge havens and inhospitable immigrant ditches. What is more, South Africa has adopted a 'quiet diplomacy' policy posture, if you will, toward Zimbabwe's millions of economic migrants and political refugees. Therefore the vast majorities of undocumented Zimbabwean refugees are deemed illegal and subject to deportation. In an analogous and markedly paradigmatic parallelism—like South Africa, the United States has adopted a rather lethargic and hushed diplomacy foreign policy toward the violent Mexican drug cartels' massacres and the long-term exodus of undocumented Mexican economic migrants into the United States. Therefore the vast majorities of undocumented Mexican migrants are deemed illegal in the U.S.A. and are subject to deportation. Furthermore, some Americans and South Africans have grown to resent the long-term encroachment of undocumented Mexican and Zimbabwean migrants into their labor markets. These xenophobic postures actively expose both of these vulnerable populations to extortion, violence, theft, municipal shakedowns, and murder.

These doppelganger-counterparts of South African and American crises can both essentially be interpreted as flawed foreign policies that fail to acknowledge political, economic, and social crises across and inside the host country's borders—coupled with a conspicuous indifference to migrants' exploitation, treatment, and protection. Dealing with the aftermath of these xenophobic attacks and violent massacres has become a daunting political caper and a social to-and-fro fluctuation in order to circumvent potential 'political landmines' in South African and United States immigration and asylum policies. This research showed instances whereby both countries made minor and major attempts to prosecute attackers, process migrants and refugee claims, protect migrants from exploitation, implement political damage control, as well as enact a variety of political and social soul-searching endeavors via adjustments in legislation, administration, dispensation, and enforcement policies.

This research has noted that migration, whether voluntary or forced, is fraught with physical, fiscal, medical, and social impediments. It involves uprooting families, leaving friends, and breaking the societal customs and values that have provided a person with a sense of continuity and self-identity. People who are smuggled or cross borders illicitly can find themselves consigned to precarious situations that threaten the physical, sexual, and/or psychological health of the migrant. Modern-day migration politics have witnessed an unmistakable hardening of attitudes and policies on immigration, and all the while undocumented migrants face more and more unstable health and social environs.

While this research did not attempt to study healthcare access in host nations among recognized refugees, residents, or (foreign-born) naturalized citizens, it sought to study female migrants that are considered undocumented, forced, or illegal immigrants without legal migration status in either South Africa (Zimbabwean migrants) or U.S.A. (Mexican migrants) who have sought emergency health care. Therefore there was a manifest need to address specific international, regional, and/or national laws and treatises that addressed their rights to asylum and healthcare access, including local (state), regional, federal, and international treatises; the beneficial and negative pushes and pulls of migration; policy enforcement and litigation;

gender-based asylum jurisprudence cases; and a few current and future trends in South African and American policy development vis-à-vis healthcare rights, asylum, enforcement, and litigation.

Our interviews uncovered that some Zimbabwean patients are denied care, charged exorbitant and usury fees, subjected to long delays, extortion, and/or improper healthcare treatment, or prematurely discharged—making health care unrealizable for many migrants. These policies not only reflect a violation of medical ethics, but a violation of the South African Constitution. The government of South Africa must do more to confirm that hospitals and clinic healthcare staff is cognizant and mindful about the rights of refugees, asylum-seekers, and migrants to access the RSA public health system, regardless of their legal status. Our research also showed that Mexican migrant's access to America's high-cost, high-tech emergency health care is fiscally out of bounds. Though it was noted that any American healthcare's denial of treatment or mistreatment is kept in check, to some degree, due to the hyper-litigious American environ and easy access to lawyers and advocacy groups (who will sue on behalf of the plaintiff for malpractice, revocation of licensure, and civil and/or criminal litigation).

Migration can either provide a constructive economic and social impact through a vibrant labor force, and rich cultural communities, or it can assert negative effects such as human trafficking, labor exploitation, and welfare and healthcare fraud. Most typically, migration produces both good and bad corollaries. Immigration policies in the United States and South Africa should be considered as critical and paramount to its citizenry as federally mandated education, health care, and defense stratagems. What seems sorely lacking is the establishment of adequate and data-comparable evaluation systems that would execute and facilitate all stages of policy formation and implementation. What is certain is that immigration and asylum policies cannot be evaluated solely via economic terms when there are numerous human rights, international security, public health, education, and national identity issues that must be weighed and kept in a delicate balance. Moreover, migration policies should stop ascertaining their effectiveness based solely on a high-income country's own national interest, but rather approach migration and asylum policy as intertwined regional and global policies that affect employment, education, foreign affairs, development, and healthcare access. There remains a great potential for courts and international conventions to improve fair access within each country's system and to decrease inequalities through the interpretation of existing legislation in both of these jurisdictions. Each nation's willingness to do so hinges on the country's ongoing commitment and conviction in their role concerning the public's access to emergency health care.

In sweeping biological terms, women suffer from many of the same diseases and illnesses as men—but they endure them uniquely as women within their unique physiological and psychosocial variations and contexts. Current research points to increasing exposures and losses in disasters and refugee emergencies, with impacts becoming demonstrably more pronounced due to ongoing social, political, and economic issues that dramatically and adversely affect women's health care. According to the previously mentioned research, the study of sex-based health differences can yield greater insight into understanding biological disease mechanisms, which can lead to improved treatments and outcomes. The study of more effective treatments and outcomes among female refugees and forced migrants, like Mexican and Zimbabwean women, constructs a critical dimension to addressing women's health needs in their host and home countries. However, how all of these complexities in gender-based biology may be applied and implemented into more effective and pro-active female refugee care and post-disaster settings have yet to be categorically researched, defined, and determined. As we've discussed, current research points to increasing exposures and losses in disasters, with impacts becoming demonstrably more pronounced due to ongoing social, political, and economic issues that dramatically and adversely affect women's health care. So when we fail to effectively address gender-based healthcare policies, we can trigger an impending environment rampant with unnecessary suffering, disabilities, and slower recoveries for female forced migrants and disaster victims. We have seen in these reports that women suffer from many of the same diseases and illnesses as men, yet they endure them uniquely as women. Today's gender-based disaster/forced migration/refugee EMS research should not only seek to identify problems, but emphasize feasible interventions which could significantly reduce pain, suffering, and long-term post-disaster care costs. Gender-based EMS awareness combined with the application of effective supplies, services, and interventions will allow planners and providers to take a more cognizant and proactive (as opposed to reactive) approach to gender-specific needs assessment, care, and advocacy. As an emergency care provider, I have a duty to assist all patients, and this includes to fight against the marginalization of women in refugee emergency healthcare planning and provision programs. Indeed today it is no longer a question of whether women have gender-distinctive healthcare concerns and needs during and after disasters, and in relief efforts—it's a question how we can research, recognize, and react to these differences, and impart equity, access, and more effective treatment for undocumented women in emergency health care.

This research undertook a small sampling of one-on-one interviews with the rationale that a gender-specific focus could help to identify and establish particular gender-based differences in the treatment, behaviors, opportunities, and vulnerabilities of undocumented and forced migrant females that have sought out emergency health care. This information should lay some groundwork for future research, and also assist emergency healthcare planners and providers to adequately plan for women in future forced migration scenarios and disasters. The interviews queried women on six dimensions of their emergency healthcare experience. The questions were targeted to ascertain each woman's role as a decision-maker in seeking emergency medical care; barriers to obtaining care; assessment of accessibility, availability, quality, equity, and credibility of care; usage of the services; assessment of provider response; and gender-equitable treatment throughout the process. According to this research's small snowball random sampling of 10–14 women from each country, the undocumented Zimbabwean women in Johannesburg sought out emergency care 16 times more than their Mexican female counterparts in Houston, Texas. While the interviewed Zimbabwean women totaled an average of five visits, the interviewed Mexican women averaged a mere two visits, even though the Mexican women's length of stay was eight times longer at an average of almost seven years in the host nation. Since the median age of the women interviewed was 32, the majority of the women fell within child-bearing ages, so the use of obstetrical care was not unexpected, with half utilizing obstetrical/gynecological (OB/GYN) services. The type of emergency health care that was sought out by both of these groups of women proved rather analogous within the specific areas of obstetrical care, dental care, and hypertension (high blood pressure). Of particular note was the variation in the cited illness' acuity and communicability/ infectious nature. More infectious communicable diseases (TB and HIV) were cited by Zimbabwean females (at less than one-fourth), than their Mexican Latina counterparts at 1 out of 10. Plus, half of the interviewed Mexican women cited non-acute illnesses, such as diarrhea, flu, migraines, etc., compared to (less than one-fourth) of the Zimbabwean women. From a fiscal and public healthcare perspective, the tremendous distinction between higher-cost, long-term communicable infectious diseases and low acuity minor illnesses (short-term and less costly) cannot be disregarded. Yet perhaps the most surprising finding was the significantly high number of Mexican women, 6 out of 10, who cited depression as one of their indications for seeking emergency health care. Nonetheless, it is meaningful to note that 100% of the Mexican women who reported domestic abuse also had cited depression as the one (or the only) illness that they sought medical attention for in the U.S.A. One female had even sought out emergency medical attention due to physical trauma inflicted by her abusive spouse. This is a significant finding in that domestic abuse can lead to physical trauma, emotional turmoil, and depression.

This study also uncovered key concerns in emergency healthcare services, including in several cases the careless (or even medically negligent) execution of emergency triage and patient assessment protocols. While life-saving patient care seemingly hung in the balance on the inconstant dispositions of receiving clerks in some aforementioned public Johannesburg hospitals—this same xenophobic exasperation and prejudiced nationalist frustration was also intermittently aimed at other perceived "foreigners" in the United States as well. In essence, what the interviews uncovered was the gaping chasm between theoretical healthcare rights and the practical effects of those rights. Most notably, in America the Mexican women could ill afford sky-high medical costs and this undermined their trust in the all-too profitable "business" side of America's 'wallet biopsy' health care—constructing scarcely surmountable fiscal barriers to health care. Undocumented Mexican's health care in Houston and throughout the United States is predominantly framed by socio-economic factors such as language and cultural barriers, lack of access to preventive care, and a lack of health insurance. However, language fluency does widely fluctuate among the heterogeneous Hispanic subgroups who reside within the mainland U.S. borders. Meanwhile, in South Africa, the Zimbabwean women's experiences uncovered blatant xenophobic denials of care combined with a deep mistrust of the country's medical institutions and personnel—constructing physical and psychological barriers to health care. Hence the day-to-day reality of many forced migrants' experiences in claiming their accorded healthcare rights in Johannesburg- and Houston-based emergency rooms was proven to be more theoretical than practical in its distribution and disposition.

One tediously persistent notion among relief agencies and organizations can be to view women as ill-fated victims, rather than focusing on efforts that build upon women's strengths in refugee and forced migration scenarios. But disaster reconstruction efforts can bring about opportunities to transform prior inequalities, and an auspicious hypothesis is that these post-disaster changes in gender roles can provide women a more equitable share of real community power and a heightened social status. Even though this particular piece of research and its interviews does not directly address women's post-migration roles, it may help prepare the path for more such research to be undertaken. Therefore in order to affect gender-based policies that work, EMS and disaster planning need to offer women supplies and services that alleviate both the short-term impacts and long-term effects on this population's overall health prognoses. To that end, I compiled a 20-point "Gender-Aware Disaster Care" checklist of provisions, services, and aids that explicitly help to address and reduce impact, acuity, and costs in post-disaster healthcare provisioning, which included: high gender input throughout all stages of planning, preparedness, response, recovery, and reconstruction efforts; a women's 'Principal Point of Contact' Resource Area; private, enclosed OB/GYN assessment, and care area; daily prenatal nutritional advocacy; a pregnancy registry; training to effectively triage pregnant women; "stress-free zone" breastfeeding area for lactating women; sterile delivery kits; rape intake provisioning;

prenatal vitamins (folic acid and ferrous sulfate supplements); pregnancy testing supplies, ultrasound, and OB/GYN services; sexually transmitted disease (STD) testing, information, and treatment; breastfeeding supplies and on-site lactation consultants; a 'fact sheet' of information to all pregnant and lactating women on potential effects of vaccines, environmental toxins, and exposures on pregnancies and outcomes; a 'fact sheet' to women and girls on all relevant information concerning post-disaster onset, symptoms, and treatment of potential vaginal infections, genital rashes, environmental contamination, and toxic shock syndrome; a variety of contraception; feminine hygiene kits; make female gynecologists and physicians available in areas where religious/patriarchal/social traditions limit or prohibit non-female physical and/or pelvic exams for women; antifungal yeast infection and genital rash products; and offer a wide variety (of all sizes) in clean female undergarments. It can be hypothesized that the stockpiling and provision of these gender-aware supplies and services could serve to decrease the risk for adverse pregnancy and infant outcomes, recurrent healthcare costs and concerns, as well as reducing requirements for multiple medical interventions (ER visits, physician care, etc.).

Forced migration, disaster research, and practices in emergency management are increasingly focusing on reducing the social vulnerability of at-risk population groups, sometimes referred to as Disaster Risk Reduction, (known as DRR in social-science circles). This paradigm shift requires an increased understanding of the social, political, and economic factors that generate vulnerabilities to hazards and form the differential abilities of these at-risk populations to survive and make adaptations that can reduce their risks. It should, in my opinion, also seek to encompass a more perceptive and proactive (rather than reactive) acumen into how policy decisions by local, state, and federal governments and healthcare providers can be reformed in order to better facilitate more efficacious public health measures, gender sensitivity, resiliency, and adaptive risk responses.

FACING FORWARD

As a final point, some healthcare experts, political and social scientists, and researchers may argue that these previously cited issues need only be 'retrofitted' with former examples of ad-hoc political gestures—gestures worth no more than temporary Band-Aids—without instituting any contemporary, long-term, or enforceable social, fiscal, and political resolutions. However, this research contends that it is critical for countries to reexamine its most rudimentary, fundamental suppositions about its national emergency health care: How it is to be defined, how it is to be financed, its accountability to women, and finally—its correlation to supply and demand between documented residents and undocumented forced migrants and 'illegal' refugees. Without the overhaul and efficacious dissemination of this primary national assessment, the secondary- and tertiary-level (state, regional, local, etc.) healthcare remodel has little hope to be implemented or enforced. However, over time, the continued mass movement of Zimbabwean and Mexican forced migrants (and other refugees) may force the need for broad immigration reform and precipitate a reconsideration of U.S. and South African asylum policies, politics, and procedures. Whether welcome or not by immigration hardliners, these mass migrations will precipitate the need to adjust the asylum system in order to more effectively deal with twenty-first century asylum-seekers.

Demonstrably, time is of the essence in establishing gender-based EMS policies, particularly in light of the serious threat of the Ebola hemorrhagic virus, Cholera, and avian bird flu pandemics, and escalating impacts of natural disasters through climate change and population growth. This research has demonstrated that women have unique and gender-distinctive physical, psychological, social, and economic needs, as well as unique vulnerabilities and opportunities in disasters. It has also attempted to give voice to the outrage of inequities, injustices, and inhumanities in undocumented women's emergency healthcare access as witnessed through my firsthand experiences as a frontline activist, political social scientist, and international aid worker. It is my opinion that women continue to be an overlooked and underutilized (but vital) part of every community's forced migration/refugee emergency response effort—whether they act in their traditional roles or transcend them. No longer can women, who make up the silent majority of the world's poor, be relegated to the *womenandchildren* catch-all classification of former disaster mitigation, emergency healthcare aid response, refugee and forced migration recovery programs.

This research has attempted to not only identify these relevant post-disaster issues, but to emphasize interventions like female-specific supplies and services, needs assessments, crises support interventions, networking, and advocacy. The suppositions of this research indicate that in emergency and forced migration/refugee healthcare management, it is better to plan *with* women—rather than *for* them. Planning with less than half of a community (i.e. men only) can only lead to further misconceptions as to how to most effectively meet women's gender-specific needs. When emergency, refugee/forced migration, aid and development programs fail to empower women—they fail to empower the community. Fundamentally, gender equity in disaster planning and aid is densely rooted in social, health care, and human rights justice affairs. This work aspires to bridge the current chasm of gender-disaggregated data, helping to uncover gender-based behavioral differences and harness those missed opportunities in women's undocumented forced migration disaster EMS planning, mitigation, response, and recovery.

Unless both the 'sending' and 'receiving' nations work in concert to address forced migration and refugee action in a way that esteems principles of international cooperation, human dignity, and the right to lifesaving emergency health care for all—there will remain grievous social injustices and reprehensible offenses to public health. In the end, if we are to effectively engage in the struggle for equitable emergency health care as a human right, we must proactively meet the emergency healthcare needs of undocumented women by closing political loopholes, eradicating prejudicial and xenophobic institutionalized healthcare policies, and enforcing regulations that will change today's theoretical healthcare rights into tomorrow's tangible practices.

Appendix A

Gender, Justice, and Health Questionnaire

Both the participant information and informal consent (A&B) areas are to be read aloud to potential participants prior to the participant's invitation to participate in research.

A) Participant Information:
Hello, I'm Roxane Richter and I'm a Ph.D. student at the University of the Witwatersrand. With these questions, I'm researching women's experiences as an undocumented migrant accessing emergency healthcare. I would like to ask you some questions on your experiences getting, or trying to get, emergency medical care in ________ (U.S.A./RSA). I'm trying to see what kind of an experience you had getting to healthcare services when you needed them in this country.

The interview should take about 10–20 minutes and I won't ask your name or any personal information about where you live or work, etc., so no one can identify you in my written research paper. You can answer some of the questions or none at all—it's all your choice and nothing will happen. We can stop whenever you want to and if you feel upset or ill, you can tell me and we'll stop, okay?

- Have you (yourself) tried to get emergency care? (if "yes," then proceed)
- Is this a comfortable place for you to speak? (if "yes," then proceed)
- Do you have any questions for me? (if "no," then proceed)

B) Verbal Informed Consent:

- If you agree to answer some or all of these questions, do you understand that there will not any be payment or treatment? (if "yes," then . . .)

- Do you understand that there won't be any problems or penalty if you stop or decide not to participate? (if "yes," then . . .)
- Do you have any questions for me? (if 'no,' then . . .)
- Would you like to participate? (if "yes," then . . .)

Thank you for your time.

GENDER, SOCIAL JUSTICE & HEALTH QUESTIONNAIRE

1. I am _____ years old. (*must be over 18)*
2. I am ☐ Single/Divorced; ☐ Married; ☐ Widowed; ☐ Living with Partner.
3. I have ______ (these many) people live with me in my house.
4. I have _______ (these many) children (under 18 years old).
5. I also take care of other people, my ☐ brother ☐ sister ☐ grandparent ☐ sick family member ☐ nephew/cousin/niece ☐ grandchild ☐ other How many?______. Specify relationships ________________________
6. How many times have you been sick/hurt and had medical help in hospital or clinic?_______ in (these many) ____months or ____years.
7. Was it an ☐ injury = (I was hurt) or ☐ an illness = (I was sick)?
8. If you have been sick or hurt and had medical help, please explain what happened: ____

   ____
   ____
   ____
   ____
   ____
   ____
   ____
   ____
   ____
9. Please check why YOU got medical help:
   ☐ I had to go to the hospital (name):____________________ specify ☐-emergency room or ☐-surgery
   ☐ I went to a (name) clinic _________________________ or NGO __
   ____
   ☐ I went to the doctor—I was sick:
      ☐ Fever—high temperature
      ☐ Vomit—throw up
      ☐ Diarrhea
      ☐ Body weakness
      ☐ Headache

- ☐ Cough
- ☐ Other: Specify: ______________________________

☐ I was pregnant, so I had to see a doctor (*obstetrical*)
☐ I had female problems (discharge, bleeding—*gynecological*)
☐ Teeth hurt—dentist
☐ Skin rash or itch (*dermatological*)
☐ I have a disease, it is ______________________________
☐ Trouble breathing (*respiratory*)
☐ I have high blood pressure or ☐ diabetes
☐ I needed medicine for ______________________________
☐ Trouble with eyes: (*ophthalmic* ☐ vision) or (*optometry* ☐ eyeglasses)
☐ I was feeling bad—panic attack, depression, mental health counsel/issue
☐ I was raped
☐ I was hurt: ☐ in an accident; ☐ by another person; other ________
☐ Other: ______________________________

10. How far did you have to travel to get medical help? ________ kilometers
11. How much did you have to pay for the medical help? ____________
12. Are you better now—healed, healthy? ☐ Yes or ☐ No. If no, why are you not? ______________________________
13. In the clinic/hospital, people were nice and good to me: ☐ Yes ☐ No
14. In the clinic/hospital, I got very good help and medicine: ☐ Yes ☐ No
15. In the clinic/hospital, I got all the medicines and help I wanted: ☐ Yes ☐ No
16. Did you ever need medicine or help, but not get any? Why? ________
____
____
17. What are the problems for you to get help when you are sick or hurt?
☐ No money
☐ No hospital or clinic
☐ The hospital, doctor, or clinic is too far away
☐ I am scared of hospital and doctors or ☐ I don't trust hospitals, doctors
☐ I am scared of government
☐ Taboo—people will think I am sick or weak or I will make them sick, too
☐ My husband or family said, "NO, you cannot go!"
18. While you were in this other foreign country, did you ever:
☐ Feel threatened—Worry for your safety?
☐ Feel afraid because ______________________________
☐ Things were stolen from me
☐ Husband hurt me

☐ Someone hurt me . . . ☐ sexual/harass . . . or ☐ physical; beat me
Please explain: ____
____
____

19. As a woman, are there problems for you to ask and get help when you are sick or hurt? Explain:____________________________________
____
____

20. Sometimes when people move to another country, people have trouble sleeping, or feel sad—What kind of feelings did you have when you moved into country and how have they changed now?______________
____
____
____

21. Race: ___ African ___ Hispanic ___ Asian ___ Bi-Racial ___ Other
22. How many years did you go to school?___________________________
23. How many years have you been in foreign country? _______________

THANK YOU for Your Time!

Appendix B

Zvemamiriro edu, Zvemitemo NeZveutano Mibvunzo neMhinduro

Zviri mugwaro iri chibvumirano cheari kubvunzwa uchaverengwa kwaari kana anoverenga pachake mibvunzo isati yatanga.

A) Chiziviso kune ari kubvunzwa:
Mhoroi, Ndinonzi Roxane Richter uye ndiri mudzidzi wePH.D. paUniversity yeWitwatersrand. Nemibvunzo iyi, ndiri kutsvaga zvinosangana nevanhukadzi vanobva kunyika yeMexico vachigara zvisiri pamitemo muUSA. Ndino kukubvunzai mibvunzo yezvamunosangana nazvo kana muchida, kana kuwana rubatsiro rwekurapwa muUSA. Ndiri kuda kunyatsoona zvawakasangana nazvo pawaida kuwana rubatsiro rwekurapwa munyika ino.

Kubvunzwa mibvunzo iyi kunotora nguva inoita maminitsi gumi kusvika gumi nemashanu uye handibvunze zita rako uye zveupenyu hwako maererano kwaunogara kana kushanda nezvimwe. Hapana anokwanisa kukuziva mugwaro rangu iri. Unokwanisa kupindura imwe mibvunzo kana kuregera – Isarudzo yako uye hapana chinoitika.

- Wakamboda kuwana rubatsiro rwekurapwa here muno munyika yeUSA? (kana ari "hongu," enderera mberi)
- Uri kugara zvisiri pamutemo munyika iyi? (kana ari "hongu," enderera mberi) . . . .

B) Kubvuma kwako:

- Kana uchinge wabvuma kupindura imwe mibvunzo kana yese zvayo, unowirirana nazvo here kuti hapana mubhadharo? (kana ari "hongu," enderera mberi . . .)

- Unonzwisisa here kuti hapana dambudziko kana mhosva kana uchinge waramba kana kuzoramba kuenderera mberi? (kana ari "hongu," enderera mberi . . .)
- Uri kuda here kupindura mibvunzo? (kana ari "hongu," enderera mberi . . .)

Tinotenda nenguva yako.

ZVEMAMIRIRO EDU, ZVEMITEMO NEZVEUTANO MIBVUNZO NEMHINDURO

1. Ndine makore _____ ekuberekwa. (*Unofanira wapfura makore gumi nesere ekuberekwa)*
2. Ndiri ☐ Musikana/Ndakasiyana nemurume; ☐ Ndakaroorwa; ☐ Ndiri Shirikadzi; ☐ Ndiri kugara nemurume.
3. Ndine ______ (vakawanda sei) vanhu vari kugara neni mumba mangu.
4. Ndine _______ (vakawanda sei) vana (vari pasi pemakore gumi nesere ekuberekwa).
5. Ndinochengeta vamwe vanhu ava vanoti, ☐ hanzvadzi ☐ mukoma/ munininа ☐ ambuya/sekuru?hama inorwara ☐ muzukuru ☐ muzukuru ☐ nevamwe Vakawanda sei?______. Nyatsotsanangura ukama hwacho ____________________________
6. Wakamborwara kana kukuvara kakawanda zvakadii uye wakabatsirwa muchiptara chikuru here kana chidiki?_______ mu (zvakawanda sei) . . . ____ mwedzi kana ____ makore.
7. Wanga ☐ wakuvara kana ☐ chirwere = (ndairwara)?
8. Kana wakakuvara kana kurwara uye ukarapwa, ndinokumbira kuti unyatsotsanangura zvakaitika:

   ____
   ____
   ____
   ____
   ____
   ____
   ____
   ____
   ____

9. Ongorora kuti sei wakawana rubatsiro rwekurapwa:
   ☐ Ndakaenda kuchipatara chikuru(zita rechipatara): ______________
   ☐-Munosvikira varwere kana ☐-Munovhiyirwa varwere kana kumwe
   ____
   ☐ Ndakaenda (zita) kuchipatara chidiki

☐ Ndakaenda kwachiremba – Ndairwara:
  ☐ Kupisa miviri
  ☐ Kurutsa
  ☐ Kuita manyoka
  ☐ Kuneta muviri
  ☐ Kurwara nemusoro
  ☐ Kukosora
  ☐ Zvimwe: Nyatsotsanangura: ________________________

☐ Ndaiva nenhumbu, saka ndakanoona chiremba (*zvevanenhumbu*)

☐ Ndairwara nezvevanhukadzi (kuburitsa ropa-zvevakadzi)

☐ Mazino airwadza – Chiremba wemazino

☐ Chirwere cheganda kana kuvava (*zvemakanda*)

☐ Ndine chirwere, chinonzi ______________________________

☐ Ndinonetseka kufema (*zvekufema*)

☐ Ndine High blood pressure kana ☐ Chirwere chesugar

☐ Ndaida mushonga we ________________________________

☐ Ndinonetseka ne maziso; (zvemaziso ☐-kuona) kana (*zvekuita nemaziso* ☐-zvekuonesa)

☐ Ndaisanzwa zvakanaka – kuvhunduka, kusuruwara, kubatsirwa zvekurwara nepfungwa

☐ Ndakabatwa chibharo

☐ Ndaka kuvara: ☐ munjodzi; ☐ kukuvadzwa nemumwe munhu; ___

☐ Zvimwe: ______________________________________

10. Wakafamba nzvimbo yakareba sei kuti uwane rubatsiro rwekurapwa? ______________ mamaera
11. Waka bhadhariswa mari yakawanda sei mukurapwa kwako? _______
12. Wavakunzwa sei – wakapora, wave neutano here? ☐ Hongu kana ☐ Kwete . . . Kana ari kwete, sei uri kudaro? _________________
13. Muchipatara chidiki/chihombe vanhu vaiva vakanaka kwandiri: ☐ Hongu ☐ Kwete
14. Muchipatara chidiki/chihombe ndakawana, rubatsiro rwakanaka nemishonga: ☐ Hongu ☐ Kwete
15. Michipatara chidiki/chihombe, ndakawana mishonga yose nerubatsiro rwandaida: ☐ Hongu ☐ Kwete
16. Une musi here wawaida mishonga kana rubatsiro asi ukashaya zvose? Zvakadaro sei?______________________________________

    ____

    ____
17. Ndeapi matambudziko aunosangana nawo kuwana rubatsiro uchinge warwara kana kukuvara?

    ☐ Kushaya mari

    ☐ Kushaya chipatara chihombe kana chidiki

- ☐ Chipatara chihombe, chiremba, kana chipatara chidiki zviri kure
- ☐ Ndinotya zvipatara, chiremba kana? Handina chivimbo nezvipatara kana ana chiremba
- ☐ Ndinotya hurumende
- ☐ Zvinofungwa nevamwe kuti kana ndiri murwere ndinokonzera kuti varwarewo
- ☐ Murume wangu kana mhuri yangu yakati, KWETE, hausi kuzoenda!

18. Pawakange uri imwe nyika isiri yako,wakambosangana neizvi :
    - ☐ Kutyisidzirwa – Kutyira hupenyu wako?
    - ☐ Kutya pamusana pe ________________________________
    - ☐ Zvinhu zvawakabirwa.
    - ☐ Murume wako akakukuvadza
    - ☐ Kukuvadzwa nemumwe . . . ☐ kubatwa chibharo/ kunetswa . . . kana ☐ kubatwa muviri; kurohwa
    - ☐ Nyatsotsanangura: ________________________________

      ____

      ____

19. Iwe semunhukadzi, une matambudzikohere aunoda kubvunza kana kutsvaga rubatsiro uchinge warwara kana kukuvara? Tsanangura:_____

    ____

    ____

    ____

20. Kana vanhu vachienda imwe nyika, vanonetseka nokurara uye vanogara vakasurukirwa – Iwe wakanzwa sei pawakaenda imwe nyika uye wava kunzwa sei mazuva ano? ________________________________

    ____

    ____

    ____

21. Rudzi rwako: ___ WekuAfrika ___ Hispanic ___ WekuAsia ___ Rudzi Rwakasanganiswa ___ Zvimwe
22. Wakaenda kuchikoro makore mangani? ________________________
23. Wava nemakore mangani munyika isiri yekwako? ________________

TATENDA nenguva yawatipa!

Appendix C

Cuestionario de género, justicia y salud

Tanto la información participante y consentimiento verbal o informal Áreas & (b) pueden ser leer en voz alta a los posibles participantes o ser leído por el participante antes a entrevista.

A) de información de participante:
Hola, soy Roxane Richter y soy un estudiante de doctorado en la Universidad de Witwatersrand. Con estas preguntas, yo estoy investigando experiencias de la mujer como asistencia un indocumentados mexicano migrante acceso a emergencia sanitaria en los Estados Unidos. Me gustaría hacerle algunas preguntas sobre su experiencia de obtener o intentar obtener, atención médica de emergencia. que estoy tratando de ver qué tipo de una experiencia había que llegar a servicios de atención médica cuando usted necesita de ellos en este país.

La entrevista debería tomar unos 10–15 minutos y no pido su nombre o cualquier información personal acerca de donde usted vive o trabajo, etc., por lo que nadie puede identificar al usuario en mi documento de investigación escrita. Usted puede responder a algunas de las preguntas o ninguno en absoluto: es toda su elección y no pasará nada.

- Ha intentado obtener emergencia¿atención de en los Estados Unidos? (si «sí,» continúe)
- Eres unindocumentados¿migrantes? (si «sí,» continúe) . . . .

B) verbal o consentimiento informado:

- Si usted está de acuerdo responder a algunas o a todas estas preguntas, entiende usted que habrá no cualquier ser pago o tratamiento? (si "sí," continúe

- Entiende usted que no habrá problemas ni pena si dejar o no decide participar? (si "sí," continúe . . .)
- ¿Le gustaría participar? (si «sí», entonces . . .)

Gracias por su tiempo.

CUESTIONARIO DE GÉNERO, JUSTICIA Y SALUD

1. Estoy _____ años de edad. (*debe ser mayor de 18 años*)
2. Estoy ☐ Single/divorciados; ☐ Se casó con; ☐ Viudas; ☐ Viven con socios.
3. Tengo ______ (este) muchos viven conmigo en mi casa.
4. Tengo _______ (este muchos) niños (menores de 18 años de edad).
5. yo también tener cuidado de otras personas, mi ☐ hermano ☐ hermana ☐ abuelo ☐ miembro de la familia enfermo ☐ sobrino, el primo/el sobrina ☐ nieto ☐ otro cómo muchos? ______. Especificar las relaciones
6. ¿Cuántas veces ha usted enfermos/daño y había ayuda médica en el hospital o clínica? _______ en (esta muchas) . . . ____months o ____years.
7. Es un ☐ Lesión = (I was hurt) o ☐ un enfermedades = (estaba enferma)?
8. Si han sido heridos o enfermos y había ayuda médica, por favor, explicar lo que ocurrió: ____

   ____
   ____
   ____
   ____
   ____
   ____
   ____
   ____
   ____
9. Por favor compruebe por qué usted obtuvo ayuda médica:
   - ☐ Tuve que ir a la hospital (nombre): ____________________ ☐-Sala de emergencias o ☐-cirugía u otros ____________________
   - ☐ Fui a un ________________________ de clínica de (nombre)
   - ☐ fui al médico – estaba enferma:
     - ☐ Fiebre alta temperatura
     - ☐ Vómito vómito en
     - ☐ Diarrea
     - ☐ Debilidad del cuerpo
     - ☐ Dolor de cabeza

- ☐ Tos
- ☐ Otros: especificar: ______________________________

☐ estaba embarazada, por lo que tenía que ver a un médico (*obstetricia*)
☐ tuve problemas femeninos (descarga, sangrado – *ginecológicos*)
☐ Dienteslastimar – dentista
☐ Erupciones en la piel o prurito (*Dermatología*)
☐ Tengo una enfermedad, es ______________________________
☐ Dificultad para respirar (*respiratorias*)
☐ tengo presión arterial alta o ☐ Diabetes
☐ Necesitaba medicina para ______________________________
☐ Problemas con los ojos; (*oftálmica* ☐ -visión) o (*Optometría* ☐ -gafas)
☐ me sentí mal – pánico de ataque, la depresión, el abogado/problema de salud mental
☐ Yo fui violada
☐ estaba herido: ☐ en un accidente; ☐ por otra persona; o tros _____
☐ Other: ______________________________

10. Hasta qué punto ¿tienes a viajar para obtener ayuda médica? millas de ______________________________
11. ¿Cuánto tienes que pagar por la ayuda médica? ______________
12. ¿Son mejor ahora – curado, saludable? ☐ sí o ☐ No . . . If no, por qué usted no son? ______________________________
13. En el hospital/clínica, personas eran agradable y buena para mí: ☐ Sí ☐ N
14. En el hospital/clínica, tengo muy buena ayuda y medicina: ☐ Sí ☐ N
15. En el hospital/clínica, tengo todos los medicamentos y ayuda quería: ☐ Sí ☐ N
16. ¿Nunca necesita medicamentos o ayuda, pero no obtener cualquiera? Por qué? ______________________________
____
____
17. ¿Cuáles son los problemas para que usted obtenga ayuda cuando usted está enfermo o herido?
    ☐ Sin dinero
    ☐ Ningún hospital o clínica
    ☐ El hospital, el médico o la clínica está demasiado lejos
    ☐ estoy asustado de hospital y médicos o ☐ No confío en hospitales, los médicos
    ☐ Tengo miedo del Gobierno
    ☐ Tabú: la gente se piensa estoy enfermo o débil o les enfermos, haré emasiado
    ☐ Mi marido o de la familia dijo, "NO, no puede ir"!

18. Mientras estabas en este otro país extranjero, ha nunca:
    - ☐ Se sienten amenazados–Worry para su seguridad?
    - ☐ Sentir miedo porque ________________________________
    - ☐ Las cosas fueron robadas de me
    - ☐ Marido herido me
    - ☐ Alguien herido me&csexual/harass . . . o cfísica; batirme
    - ☐ Por favor explicar: ________________________________
19. ¿Como mujer, hay problemas para poder pedir y obtener ayuda cuando usted está enfermo o herido? ____________________________

    ____

    ____
20. A veces cuando la gente se desplaza a otro país, las personas tienen problemas para dormir o sentir triste – ¿qué tipo de sentimientos, ¿ha ha cuando se trasladó a país, y cómo ellos cambiaron ahora? __________

    ____

    ____

    ____
21. ___ Africano hispanos ___ Asia ___ BI-racial de la raza: otros
22. ¿Cuántos años ir a la escuela? ____________________________
23. ¿Cuántos años ha estado en país extranjero? __________________

Appendix D

The Patients' Rights Charter – South Africa

For many decades the vast majority of the South African population has experienced either a denial or violation of fundamental human rights, including rights to health care services. To ensure the realization of the right of access to health care services as guaranteed in the Constitution of the Republic of South Africa (Act No 108 of 1996), the Department of Health is committed to upholding, promoting and protecting this right and therefore proclaims this PATIENTS' RIGHTS CHARTER as a common standard for achieving the realization of this right. This Charter is subject to the provisions of any law operating within the Republic of South Africa and to the financial means of the country.

A Healthy and Safe Environment

Everyone has the right to a healthy and safe environment that will ensure their physical and mental health or well-being, including adequate water supply, sanitation, and waste disposal as well as protection from all forms of environmental danger, such as pollution, ecological degradation, or infection.

Participation in Decision-Making

Every citizen has the right to participate in the development of health policies and everyone has the right to participate in decision-making on matters affecting one's health.

Access to Healthcare

Everyone has the right of access to health care services that include:

i. receiving timely emergency care at any healthcare facility that is open regardless of one's ability to pay;
ii. treatment and rehabilitation that must be made known to the patient to enable the patient to understand such treatment or rehabilitation and the consequences thereof;
iii. provision for special needs in the case of newborn infants, children, pregnant women, the aged, disabled persons, patients in pain, person living with HIV or AIDS patients;
iv. counseling without discrimination, coercion, or violence on matters such as reproductive health, cancer, or HIV/AIDS;
v. palliative care that is affordable and effective in cases of incurable or terminal illness;
vi. a positive disposition displayed by healthcare providers that demonstrate courtesy, human dignity, patience, empathy, and tolerance; and
vii. health information that includes the availability of health services and how best to use such services and such information shall be in the language understood by the patient.

Knowledge of One's Health Insurance/Medical Aid Scheme

A member of a health insurance or medical aid scheme is entitled to information about that insurance or medical aid scheme and to challenge, where necessary, the decisions of such health insurance or medical aid scheme relating to the member.

Choice of Health Services

Everyone has the right to choose a particular healthcare provider for services or a particular health facility for treatment provided that such choice shall not be contrary to the ethical standards applicable to such healthcare providers or facilities, and the choice of facilities in line with prescribed service delivery guide lines.

Be Treated by a Named Healthcare Provider

Everyone has the right to know the person that is providing health care and therefore must be attended to by clearly identified healthcare providers.

Confidentiality and Privacy

Information concerning one's health, including information concerning treatment may only be disclosed with informed consent, except when required in terms of any law or an order of the court.

Informed Consent

Everyone has the right to be given full and accurate information about the nature of one's illnesses, diagnostic procedures, the proposed treatment, and the costs involved, for one to make a decision that affects anyone of these elements.

Refusal of Treatment

A person may refuse treatment and such refusal shall be verbal or in writing provided that such refusal does not endanger the health of others.

Be Referred for a Second Opinion

Everyone has the right to be referred for a second opinion on request to a health provider of one's choice.

Continuity of Care

No one shall be abandoned by a health care professional worker or a health facility which initially took responsibility for one's health.

Complain about Health Services

Everyone has the right to complain about health care services and to have such complaints investigated and to receive a full response on such investigation.

Every patient or client has the following responsibilities:

- to advise the healthcare providers on his or her wishes with regard to his or her death;
- to comply with the prescribed treatment or rehabilitation procedures;
- to enquire about the related costs of treatment and/or rehabilitation and to arrange for payment;
- to take care of health records in his or her possession;
- to take care of his or her health;
- to care for and protect the environment;
- to respect the rights of other patients and health providers;
- to utilize the healthcare system properly and not abuse it;
- to know his or her local health services and what they offer; and
- to provide healthcare providers with the relevant and accurate information for diagnostic, treatment, rehabilitation or counselling purposes.

Appendix E

U.S. Department of Health and Human Services "Fact Sheet"–For Patient Bill of Rights, 1999

THE PATIENTS' BILL OF RIGHTS IN MEDICARE AND MEDICAID

On March 26, 1997, President Clinton created the Advisory Commission on Consumer Protection and Quality in the Health Care Industry and charged it with recommend[ing] such measures as may be necessary to promote and assure health care quality and value and protect consumers and workers in the health care system. As part of that charge, the President asked the Commission to develop a "Patients' Bill of Rights" in health care.

In February 1998, President Clinton directed the Department of HHS, along with the departments of Labor, Defense, and Veterans' Affairs and the Office of Personnel Management, to use their regulatory and administrative authority to bring their health programs into compliance with the Bill of Rights and Responsibilities.

HHS' Health Care Financing Administration (HCFA) has begun the work to establish new requirements for managed care plans participating in the Medicare program. It is also working to strengthen protections for beneficiaries enrolled in Medicaid managed care. In November 1998, HHS issued a report to the Vice President showing that it is moving aggressively to strengthen existing patient protections under Medicare and Medicaid.

When these regulations are fully implemented, Medicare and Medicaid will have among the strongest patients' protections in the country. The proposed regulations give HHS a variety of monitoring and enforcement tools, including suspension of payments, civil monetary penalties, and termination from the Medicare and Medicaid programs.

BACKGROUND: THE PRESIDENT'S ADVISORY COMMISSION ON CONSUMER PROTECTION AND QUALITY IN THE HEALTH CARE INDUSTRY AND THE PATIENTS' BILL OF RIGHTS

In November 1997, President Clinton's Advisory Commission on Consumer Protection and Quality on the Health Care Industry, in an Interim Report, issued the Patients' Bill of Rights and Responsibilities. The Commission's Final Report, "Quality First: Better Health Care for All Americans," was issued in March 1998.

Co-chaired by Secretary of HHS Donna E. Shalala and Secretary of Labor Alexis M. Herman, the Commission had 34 members, including broad-based representation from consumers, businesses, labor, healthcare providers, health plans, and healthcare quality and financing experts.

The Patients' Bill of Rights and Responsibilities has three goals: to strengthen consumer confidence that the healthcare system is fair and responsive to consumer needs; to reaffirm the importance of a strong relationship between patients and their healthcare providers; and to reaffirm the critical role consumers play in safeguarding their own health. The Commission articulated seven sets of rights and one set of responsibilities:

- The Right to Information. Patients have the right to receive accurate, easily understood information to assist them in making informed decisions about their health plans, facilities and professionals.
- The Right to Choose. Patients have the right to a choice of healthcare providers that is sufficient to assure access to appropriate high-quality health care including giving women access to qualified specialists such as obstetrician-gynecologists and giving patients with serious medical conditions and chronic illnesses access to specialists.
- Access to Emergency Services. Patients have the right to access emergency health services when and where the need arises. Health plans should provide payment when a patient presents himself/herself to any ED with acute symptoms of sufficient severity "including severe pain" that a "prudent layperson" could reasonably expect the absence of medical attention to result in placing that consumer's health in serious jeopardy, serious impairment to bodily functions, or serious dysfunction of any bodily organ or part.
- Being a Full Partner in Health Care Decisions. Patients have the right to fully participate in all decisions related to their health care. Consumers who are unable to fully participate in treatment decisions have the right to be represented by parents, guardians, family members, or other conservators.

Additionally, provider contracts should not contain any so-called "gag clauses" that restrict health professionals' ability to discuss and advise patients on medically necessary treatment options.

- Care Without Discrimination. Patients have the right to considerate, respectful care from all members of the Health Care Industry at all times and under all circumstances. Patients must not be discriminated against in the marketing or enrollment or in the provision of health care services, consistent with the benefits covered in their policy and/or as required by law, based on race, ethnicity, national origin, religion, sex, age, current or anticipated mental or physical disability, sexual orientation, genetic information, or source of payment.
- The Right to Privacy. Patients have the right to communicate with healthcare providers in confidence and to have the confidentiality of their individually-identifiable health care information protected. Patients also have the right to review and copy their own medical records and request amendments to their records.
- The Right to Speedy Complaint Resolution. Patients have the right to a fair and efficient process for resolving differences with their health plans, healthcare providers, and the institutions that serve them, including a rigorous system of internal review and an independent system of external review.
- Taking on New Responsibilities. In a healthcare system that affords patients' rights and protections, patients must also take greater responsibility for maintaining good health.

MEDICARE AND MEDICAID COMPLIANCE WITH THE PATIENTS' BILL OF RIGHTS

While many of the protections articulated in the Bill of Rights are most relevant to individuals in managed care, such as those related to choice of providers and access to specialists, other protections such as complaints and appeals apply to beneficiaries not enrolled in managed care.

Medicare covers nearly 40 million individuals, of whom approximately 6.5 million, or 17%, are currently enrolled in managed care arrangements. Medicaid covers an estimated 40 million people, of whom about half are in a managed care arrangement for some or all of their health care at some point during a year.

HHS has moved aggressively to strengthen existing patient protections under Medicare and Medicaid. On June 26, 1998, the HCFA published an Interim Final rule establishing new requirements for managed care arrangements participating in Medicare. On September 29, 1998, HCFA published a Notice of Proposed Rulemaking (NPRM) strengthening protections for Medicaid beneficiaries enrolled in managed care arrangements. Generally, the Medicare protections became effective on or before January 1, 1999, and will be fully implemented by no later than December 31, 1999. States will be required to implement all new protections within one year from the effective date of the final regulation for Medicaid, which is expected to be issued by mid-1999.

When these regulations are fully implemented, Medicare and Medicaid will have among the strongest patients' protections in the country. Specifically, HHS has been able to come into compliance for managed care enrollees with critical patient protections such as information disclosure, access to emergency services, patient participation in treatment decisions, and complaints and appeals. These regulations also expand patients' ability to choose their healthcare providers and to have ready access to specialists.

In a few areas, however, both Medicare and Medicaid currently lack the statutory authority to achieve full compliance with the Patients' Bill of Rights. For example, current legislative authority also does not permit full implementation of the right to medical record confidentiality. HHS has, however, separately submitted a report to the Congress laying out the parameters for federal legislation to protect the confidentiality of health records. Additionally, while Medicare and Medicaid managed care enrollees are currently protected to the full extent of the Patients' Bill of Rights with regard to respect and non-discrimination, the rules that prohibit discrimination under fee-for-service address some, but not all, categories of protection and providers included in the right as recommended by the Commission.

The proposed regulations give HHS a variety of monitoring and enforcement tools including suspension of payments, civil money penalties, and termination from the Medicare and Medicaid programs. HHS will take all necessary actions to enforce the protections included in the Medicare and Medicaid regulations.

Specific Rights

Information Disclosure. Under proposed regulations, Medicare and Medicaid will require plans to provide critical information to consumers, both annually and upon request, that will enable them to make more informed choices about their health plans. Medicare's web site, www.medicare.gov, offers the "Medicare Compare" database to help beneficiaries evaluate different plans and decide which options are best, including comparative information about the quality of care provided to patients and about the level of satisfaction among patients with the care that they receive.

Choice of Providers and Plans. The Interim Final rule for Medicare and the proposed Medicaid managed care regulations assure provider network adequacy, by requiring that medically necessary services be available 24 hours a day, 7 days a week to enrollees. The Interim Final rule and the proposed rule also reflect the recommendations of the Commission by requiring that participating plans offer women access to qualified women's health specialists for routine preventive care, and provide consumers with complex or serious medical conditions an adequate number of direct access visits to specialists under a plan of treatment. As has been the case since the start of these programs, Medicare and Medicaid beneficiaries who obtain their care on a fee-for-service basis can choose any provider who agrees to participate in these programs.

Access to Emergency Services. The Interim Final rule for Medicare and the proposed regulations for Medicaid guarantee that emergency services will be covered when and where the need arises, in exact compliance with the Patients' Bill of Rights. Plans would not be permitted to require preauthorization in order for an enrollee to obtain emergency services. In addition, the regulations articulate a standard for post-stabilization services that is applicable to both Medicare and Medicaid managed care enrollees. This policy identifies the obligation of the plan to pay for care provided after an emergency situation is stabilized, particularly when the plan fails to authorize such care on a timely basis.

Participation in Treatment Decisions. The Interim Final rule for Medicare and the NPRM for Medicaid reflect existing and new policies that are consistent with this right, including information about treatment options and advance directives, physicians' financial disclosure and prohibition against "gag rules." Health plans will be required to provide patients with easily understood information and the opportunity to decide among all treatment options—including no treatment—consistent with the informed consent process. Managed care organizations and providers are required to discuss the use of advance directives, or "living wills" with patients and their families and to abide by the wishes as expressed in an advanced directive, except where state law permits a provider to conscientiously object. Physicians are required to disclose to Medicare and Medicaid any financial arrangements that create incentives for limiting care. Plans are prohibited from penalizing or otherwise restricting the ability of healthcare providers to communicate with and advise Medicare and Medicaid patients about medically-necessary treatment options.

Respect and Nondiscrimination. Under the Interim Final rule for Medicare and the proposed regulations for Medicaid, managed care enrollees are protected to the full extent of this right as articulated in the Bill of Rights, with regard to services, marketing and enrollment. Under fee-for-service, however,

Medicare and Medicaid protections against discrimination are largely a function of federal anti-discrimination rules that apply to recipients of federal funds. These rules address some, but not all, categories of protection and providers included in the Bill of Rights. As a result, the fee-for-service aspects of Medicare and Medicaid are in only partial compliance with this right.

Confidentiality of Health Information. The Interim Final regulations for Medicare and the proposed regulations for Medicaid require Medicare + Choice and Medicaid health plans to safeguard the privacy of any information that identifies a particular enrollee by ensuring that information from the plan (or copies of records) be released only to authorized individuals, that unauthorized individuals cannot gain access to or alter patient records, and that original medical records must be released only in accordance with federal or state law, court orders or subpoenas. In Medicaid, plans are required to establish procedures to address the confidentiality and privacy of minors, subject to applicable federal and state law.

While current federal laws and related regulations protect certain written records from disclosure outside of Medicare and Medicaid, such protections do not extend to all written records, nor to verbal communications between enrollees and providers. Protection of communication between patients and providers is a matter of state law, many of which do not afford the protections included in this right. Moreover, not all providers under Medicare and Medicaid are subject to federal laws on privacy. The Secretary's Privacy Recommendations to Congress (September 1997), if enacted, would bring all beneficiary information obtained by Medicare and Medicaid providers and plans, as well as the programs and their contractors, into compliance with this right as articulated in the Bill of Rights.

Complaints and Appeals. The Interim Final rule for Medicare and the proposed regulations for Medicaid managed care require establishment of meaningful processes for resolution of complaints and appeals. Similar processes already exist for resolution of disputes arising in fee-for-service settings.

Internal Appeals. Both the Interim Final rule for Medicare and the NPRM for Medicaid define rigorous standards for the establishment of internal (plan-level) appeal processes, with explicit timeframes for both prior authorizations and resolution of appeals at the plan level. Both the Medicare and Medicaid regulations establish a process for expedited review of prior authorizations and resolution of appeals by plans in emergency or urgent care situations. Extensions for both the standard and expedited timeframes are possible only under limited circumstances.

External Appeals. The Bill of Rights proposes that an appeal process include an independent system of external review, in order to ensure its fairness and accuracy. Medicare has long had this protection which includes a provision for expedited decisions in time-sensitive areas. Individuals who are dissatisfied with the determination of the independent external review entity have the right to pursue their claim for Medicare benefits further through an administrative review, including review by the Departmental Appeals Board and, ultimately, federal court.

The appeals process for Medicaid, as articulated in the NPRM, differs from the Bill of Rights in two significant ways. The Bill of Rights calls for the establishment of a sequential process of internal (plan-level) and external review. Under the proposed rule, however, states would be permitted to design their appeals systems so that individuals would appeal either sequentially or simultaneously to the state's fair hearing process, which otherwise serves as the independent external review entity. Second, the state fair hearing process, which serves a docket of programs and issues much broader than Medicaid managed care, currently has timeframes that are not consistent with the timeframes established by the NPRM for internal review by Medicaid managed care plans; in addition, there is no provision for expedited review.

Appendix F

EMTALA: Emergency Medical Treatment and Active Labor Act, 1986

42 USC § 1395dd—Examination and treatment for emergency medical conditions and women in labor

(a) Medical screening requirement
In the case of a hospital that has a hospital ED, if any individual (whether or not eligible for benefits under this subchapter) comes to the ED and a request is made on the individual's behalf for examination or treatment for a medical condition, the hospital must provide for an appropriate medical screening examination within the capability of the hospital's ED, including ancillary services routinely available to the ED, to determine whether or not an emergency medical condition (within the meaning of subsection (e)(1) of this section) exists.

(b) Necessary stabilizing treatment for emergency medical conditions and labor
(1) In general
If any individual (whether or not eligible for benefits under this subchapter) comes to a hospital and the hospital determines that the individual has an emergency medical condition, the hospital must provide either:
(A) within the staff and facilities available at the hospital, for such further medical examination and such treatment as may be required to stabilize the medical condition, or
(B) for transfer of the individual to another medical facility in accordance with subsection (c) of this section.
(2) Refusal to consent to treatment
A hospital is deemed to meet the requirement of paragraph (1)(A) with respect to an individual if the hospital offers the individual

the further medical examination and treatment described in that paragraph and informs the individual (or a person acting on the individual's behalf) of the risks and benefits to the individual of such examination and treatment, but the individual (or a person acting on the individual's behalf) refuses to consent to the examination and treatment. The hospital shall take all reasonable steps to secure the individual's (or person's) written informed consent to refuse such examination and treatment.

(3) Refusal to consent to transfer

A hospital is deemed to meet the requirement of paragraph (1) with respect to an individual if the hospital offers to transfer the individual to another medical facility in accordance with subsection (c) of this section and informs the individual (or a person acting on the individual's behalf) of the risks and benefits to the individual of such transfer, but the individual (or a person acting on the individual's behalf) refuses to consent to the transfer. The hospital shall take all reasonable steps to secure the individual's (or person's) written informed consent to refuse such transfer.

(c) Restricting transfers until individual stabilized

(1) Rule

If an individual at a hospital has an emergency medical condition which has not been stabilized (within the meaning of subsection (e)(3)(B) of this section), the hospital may not transfer the individual unless:

(A)

(i) the individual (or a legally responsible person acting on the individual's behalf) after being informed of the hospital's obligations under this section and of the risk of transfer, in writing requests transfer to another medical facility,

(ii) a physician (within the meaning of section 1395x (r)(1) of this title) has signed a certification that[1] based upon the information available at the time of transfer, the medical benefits reasonably expected from the provision of appropriate medical treatment at another medical facility outweigh the increased risks to the individual and, in the case of labor, to the unborn child from effecting the transfer, or

(iii) if a physician is not physically present in the ED at the time an individual is transferred, a qualified medical person (as defined by the Secretary in regulations) has signed a certification described in clause (ii) after a physician (as defined in section 1395x (r)(1) of this title), in consultation with the person, has made the determination described in such clause, and subsequently countersigns the certification; and

(B) the transfer is an appropriate transfer (within the meaning of paragraph (2)) to that facility.

A certification described in clause (ii) or (iii) of subparagraph (A) shall include a summary of the risks and benefits upon which the certification is based.

(2) Appropriate transfer

An appropriate transfer to a medical facility is a transfer—

(A) in which the transferring hospital provides the medical treatment within its capacity which minimizes the risks to the individual's health and, in the case of a woman in labor, the health of the unborn child;

(B) in which the receiving facility—

(i) has available space and qualified personnel for the treatment of the individual, and

(ii) has agreed to accept transfer of the individual and to provide appropriate medical treatment;

(C) in which the transferring hospital sends to the receiving facility all medical records (or copies thereof), related to the emergency condition for which the individual has presented, available at the time of the transfer, including records related to the individual's emergency medical condition, observations of signs or symptoms, preliminary diagnosis, treatment provided, results of any tests and the informed written consent or certification (or copy thereof) provided under paragraph (1)(A), and the name and address of any on-call physician (described in subsection (d)(1)(C) of this section) who has refused or failed to appear within a reasonable time to provide necessary stabilizing treatment;

(D) in which the transfer is effected through qualified personnel and transportation equipment, as required including the use of necessary and medically appropriate life support measures during the transfer; and

(E) which meets such other requirements as the Secretary may find necessary in the interest of the health and safety of individuals transferred.

(d) Enforcement

(1) Civil money penalties

(A) A participating hospital that negligently violates a requirement of this section is subject to a civil money penalty of not more than $50,000 (or not more than $25,000 in the case of a hospital with less than 100 beds) for each such violation. The provisions of section 1320a–7a of this title (other than subsections (a) and (b)) shall apply to a civil money penalty under this subparagraph in the same manner as such provisions apply with respect to a penalty or proceeding under section 1320a–7a (a) of this title.

(B) Subject to subparagraph (C), any physician who is responsible for the examination, treatment, or transfer of an individual in a participating hospital, including a physician on-call for the care of such an individual, and who negligently violates a requirement of this section, including a physician who—

(i) signs a certification under subsection (c)(1)(A) of this section that the medical benefits reasonably to be expected from a transfer to another facility outweigh the risks associated with the transfer, if the physician knew or should have known that the benefits did not outweigh the risks, or

(ii) misrepresents an individual's condition or other information, including a hospital's obligations under this section, is subject to a civil money penalty of not more than $50,000 for each such violation and, if the violation is gross and flagrant or is repeated, to exclusion from participation in this subchapter and State health care programs. The provisions of section 1320a–7a of this title (other than the first and second sentences of subsection (a) andsubsection (b)) shall apply to a civil money penalty and exclusion under this subparagraph in the same manner as such provisions apply with respect to a penalty, exclusion, or proceeding under section 1320a–7a (a) of this title.

(C) If, after an initial examination, a physician determines that the individual requires the services of a physician listed by the hospital on its list of on-call physicians (required to be maintained under section 1395cc (a)(1)(I) of this title) and notifies the on-call physician and the on-call physician fails or refuses to appear within a reasonable period of time, and the physician orders the transfer of the individual because the physician determines that without the services of the on-call physician the benefits of transfer outweigh the risks of transfer, the physician authorizing the transfer shall not be subject to a penalty under subparagraph (B). However, the previous sentence shall not apply to the hospital or to the on-call physician who failed or refused to appear.

(2) Civil enforcement

(A) Personal harm

Any individual who suffers personal harm as a direct result of a participating hospital's violation of a requirement of this section may, in a civil action against the participating hospital, obtain those damages available for personal injury under the law of the State in which the hospital is located, and such equitable relief as is appropriate.

(B) Financial loss to other medical facility

Any medical facility that suffers a financial loss as a direct result of a participating hospital's violation of a requirement of this section may, in a civil action against the participating hospital, obtain those damages available for financial loss, under the law of the State in which the hospital is located, and such equitable relief as is appropriate.

(C) Limitations on actions

No action may be brought under this paragraph more than two years after the date of the violation with respect to which the action is brought.

(3) Consultation with quality improvement organizations

In considering allegations of violations of the requirements of this section in imposing sanctions under paragraph (1) or in terminating a hospital's participation under this subchapter, the Secretary shall request the appropriate quality improvement organization (with a contract under part B of subchapter XI of this chapter) to assess whether the individual involved had an emergency medical condition which had not been stabilized, and provide a report on its findings. Except in the case in which a delay would jeopardize the health or safety of individuals, the Secretary shall request such a review before effecting a sanction under paragraph (1) and shall provide a period of at least 60 days for such review. Except in the case in which a delay would jeopardize the health or safety of individuals, the Secretary shall also request such a review before making a compliance determination as part of the process of terminating a hospital's participation under this subchapter for violations related to the appropriateness of a medical screening examination, stabilizing treatment, or an appropriate transfer as required by this section, and shall provide a period of 5 days for such review. The Secretary shall provide a copy of the organization's report to the hospital or physician consistent with confidentiality requirements imposed on the organization under such part B.

(4) Notice upon closing an investigation
The Secretary shall establish a procedure to notify hospitals and physicians when an investigation under this section is closed.

(e) Definitions

In this section:

(1) The term "emergency medical condition" means—
(A) a medical condition manifesting itself by acute symptoms of sufficient severity (including severe pain) such that the absence of immediate medical attention could reasonably be expected to result in—
(i) placing the health of the individual (or, with respect to a pregnant woman, the health of the woman or her unborn child) in serious jeopardy,
(ii) serious impairment to bodily functions, or
(iii) serious dysfunction of any bodily organ or part; or
(B) with respect to a pregnant woman who is having contractions—
(i) that there is inadequate time to effect a safe transfer to another hospital before delivery, or
(ii) that transfer may pose a threat to the health or safety of the woman or the unborn child.

(2) The term "participating hospital" means a hospital that has entered into a provider agreement under section 1395cc of this title.

(3)
(A) The term "to stabilize" means, with respect to an emergency medical condition described in paragraph (1)(A), to provide such medical treatment of the condition as may be necessary to assure, within reasonable medical probability, that no material deterioration of the condition is likely to result from or occur during the transfer of the individual from a facility, or, with respect to an emergency medical condition described in paragraph (1)(B), to deliver (including the placenta).
(B) The term "stabilized" means, with respect to an emergency medical condition described in paragraph (1)(A), that no material deterioration of the condition is likely, within reasonable medical probability, to result from or occur during the transfer of the individual from a facility, or, with respect to an emergency medical condition described in paragraph (1)(B), that the woman has delivered (including the placenta).

(4) The term "transfer" means the movement (including the discharge) of an individual outside a hospital's facilities at the direction of any person employed by (or affiliated or associated, directly or indirectly,

with) the hospital, but does not include such a movement of an individual who

(A) (A) has been declared dead, or

(B) leaves the facility without the permission of any such person.

(5) The term "hospital" includes a critical access hospital.

(f) Preemption

The provisions of this section do not preempt any State or local law requirement, except to the extent that the requirement directly conflicts with a requirement of this section.

(g) Nondiscrimination

A participating hospital that has specialized capabilities or facilities (such as burn units, shock-trauma units, neonatal intensive care units, or (with respect to rural areas) regional referral centers as identified by the Secretary in regulation) shall not refuse to accept an appropriate transfer of an individual who requires such specialized capabilities or facilities if the hospital has the capacity to treat the individual.

(h) No delay in examination or treatment

A participating hospital may not delay provision of an appropriate medical screening examination required under subsection: (a) of this section or further medical examination and treatment required under subsection (b) of this section in order to inquire about the individual's method of payment or insurance status.

(i) Whistleblower protections

A participating hospital may not penalize or take adverse action against a qualified medical person described in subsection (c)(1)(A)(iii) of this section or a physician because the person or physician refuses to authorize the transfer of an individual with an emergency medical condition that has not been stabilized or against any hospital employee because the employee reports a violation of a requirement of this section.

Bibliography

Adar, J., and Stevens, M. "Women's Health," in *Society, Health and Disease*, edited by Gilbert, L., Selikow, T., and Walker, L. 162–170. Braamfontein, South Africa: Ravan Press, 2002.

American Civil Liberties Union. "The War on Women." 2013. Accessed July 1, 2013. http://www.aclu.org/blog/tag/war-women.

African Charter on Human and Peoples' Rights. Addis Ababa: Organization of African Unity, 1981.

Agamben, G., and Daniel, R. *Homo Sacer: Sovereign Power and Bare Life*. Stanford, Calif.: Stanford University Press, 1998.

Agamben, G. "We Refugees." *Symposium: A Quarterly Journal in Modern Literatures*: 1995: 114–19.

Aggad, F., and Sidiropoulos, E. "South Africa's Tipping Point." Open Democracy. 2008. Accessed March 3, 2013.

AIDSMEDS. "What are the Symptoms and How is TB Diagnosed?" AIDSMEDS Publications. http://www.aidsmeds.com/articles/TB_6732.shtml (accessed June 1, 2012).

American College of Emergency Physicians. "Best Way to Solve ED Overcrowding is to Move Critical Patients to Appropriate Floors Faster." American College of Emergency Physicians, Washington, D.C., June 23, 2009.

American Heritage Dictionary. Public Welfare. American Heritage Publishing Company, 2013.

America's Health Insurance Plans Center for Policy and Research. "January 2010 Census Shows 10 Million People Covered by HAS/High-Deductible Health Plans." Washington, D.C.: America's Health Insurance Plans Center for Policy and Research, 2010.

Amnesty International USA. "*A fact sheet on Convention on the Elimination of All Forms of Discrimination against Women: A treaty for the Rights of Women.*" 2009. Accessed June 13, 2009. http://www.aiusa.org/women.

Bailey, R. "Emergency Department Billboard Waiting Times: A Solution to ED Overcrowding or a Deterrent to Patients?" *What's Up in Emergency Medicine?* Newsletter. Irving, Texas: Emergency Medicine Residents' Association, July, 2011.

Bassett, L. "Texas Loses Entire Women's Health Program over Planned Parenthood Law." *Huffington Post,* March 15, 2012.

BBC News. "Nelson Mandela Ambulance Broke Down on Way to Hospital." BBC News Africa, June 22, 2013.

BBC News. "Focus on Africa: South African Rape Survey Shock." United Kingdom: BBC News, June 18, 2009.

Behar, R. *The Vulnerable Observer: Anthropology That Breaks Your Heart.* Boston: Beacon Press, 1996.

Behar, R. *Translated Woman.* Boston: Beacon Press, 1993.

Bhugra, D. "Migration and Mental Illness." *Advances in Psychiatric Treatment,* 2001: 216–22.

Biehl, J., and Torben, E. *Vita Life in a Zone of Social Abandonment.* CA: University of California Press, 2005.

Bird, C. E., and Patricia, P. R. *Gender and Health: The Effects of Constrained Choices and Social Policies.* Cambridge: Cambridge University Press, 2008.

Biswas, R. "The Illness of Feminine Hygiene." *Clean & Hygiene Review.* Mumbai: Hammer Publishers, 2007.

Bobones, S. "U.S. Income Distribution: Just How Unequal?" Washington, D.C.: Inequality.org, February 14, 2012. http://inequality.org/unequal-americas-income-distribution (accessed March 2, 2013).

Bonomi, A. "Depression Caused by Domestic Abuse." *Examiner,* April 24, 2010.

Bruijns, S., Lee W., and Burch, V. C. "Effect of Introduction of Nurse Triage on Waiting Times in a South African Emergency Department." *Emergency Medical Journal,* 25 (2008): 395–97.

Brezosky, L. "U.S. Citizenship to be Checked in Event of a Storm: Agents to Watch those in the Valley who Board Buses to Flee a Hurricane." *San Antonio Express-News,* May 15, 2008.

Brock University. "Eustress Versus Distress." Ontario: Canada, 2013. Accessed on March 2, 2012. http://www.brocku.ca/health-services/health-education/stress/eustress-distress.

BuaNews. "South Africa: New EMS Stations for 2010 Tourney." *BuaNews,* March 16, 2010.

BuaNews. "South Africa: HCT Campaign Rolls Out in all Provinces." *BuaNews,* April 28, 2010.

Buekens, P., Xiong X., and Harville, E. "Hurricanes and Pregnancy." *Birth* 2006, 33(2): 91–93.

Burman, E. "Taking Women's Voices: The Psychological Politics of Feminization," *Psychology of Women Section Review,* 6(2004): 3–21.

Byrnes, J., David M., and William S. "Gender Differences in Risk Taking: A Meta-Analysis." *Psychological Bulletin,* 125(1999): 367–83.

Callaghan, W., Sonja, A. R., Jamieson, D., et al. "Health Concerns of Women and Infants in Times of Natural Disasters: lessons Learned from Hurricane Katrina." *Journal of Maternal Child Health,* 2007; 11(4): 307–11.

Campbell, D. "Why Fight: Humanitarianism, Principles, and Post-structuralism." *Millennium—Journal of International Studies*, 1998: 497–521.

Campbell, M. "Tsunami and the Silent Tide: The Invisible Challenge of Women's Health." *Journal of Family Planning and Reproductive Health Care*, 2005; 31(2): 95–97.

Cape Triage Group. *Cape Triage Score, Hospital Provider Manual.* Cape Triage Group. South Africa: University of Cape Town, 2005.

Centro Nacional de Comunicación Social (CENCOS). CENCOS and ARTICLE 19-Mexico, 60th Anniversary of the Universal Declaration of Human Rights, December 10, 2008.

Centro Nacional de Comunicación Social (CENCOS). "Violence and Press Freedom in Mexico: Still in the Line of Fire." CENCOS and Article 19-Mexico, May 10, 2011.

Chew, L., and Cavita, R. "Caught in the Storm: The Impact of Natural Disasters on Women." San Francisco: Global Fund for Women. December, 2005.

Centers for Disease Control. "Deaths: Preliminary Data for 2007." Atlanta, GA: U.S.A. National Vital Statistics Reports, CDC National Center for Health Statistics, August 19, 2009.

Centers for Disease Control. "HIV Cost Effectiveness." Atlanta, GA: U.S.A., CDC National Center for Health Statistics. http://www.cdc.gov/hiv/prevention/ongoing/costeffectiveness (accessed July 10, 2015).

Centers for Medicare and Medicaid Services. "Federal Reimbursement for Emergency Health Care for Illegal Immigrant Patients in the 2006 Fiscal Year." Washington, D.C.: U.S. Department of Health and Human Services, 2006.

Center for Strategic and International Studies. "Update: Drug-War Death Toll in Mexico Higher than Expected." Washington, D.C.: Office of the William E. Simon Chair, April 16, 2010.

Central Intelligence Agency. *World Factbook: Country Comparison Life Expectancy at Birth.* Washington, D.C.: Central Intelligence Agency, Independent U.S. Government Agency, 2010. https://www.cia.gov/library/publications/the-world-factbook/rankorder/2102rank.html (accessed June 1, 2013).

Central Intelligence Agency. *World Factbook: Zimbabwe: Economy.* Washington, D.C.: Central Intelligence Agency, Independent U.S. Government Agency, 2010. Accessed May 24, 2011. https://www.cia.gov/library/publications/the-world-factbook/geos/zi.html.

Chhibber, A. "Hazards of Nature, Risks and Opportunities for Development in South Asian Countries." World Bank Regional Conference. New Delhi, India: December 19–20, 2006.

CNN International. "September 11: A Memorial." Atlanta, GA: CNN News. http://cnn.com/SPECIAL (accessed May 2014).

CNN International. "UK PM: Zimbabwe Cholera Cases are International Emergency." Atlanta, GA: CNN News, 2008. http://edition.cnn.com/2008/WORLD/africa/12/06/zimbabwe.main/index.html (accessed January 9, 2009).

CNN International. "What in the World—Zimbabwe." Fareed Zakaria Global Public Square TV segment. Atlanta, GA: CNN News, February 3, 2013.

Collinson, M., Kubaje, A., Micheal, W., and Sally, F., (Eds.). "The Dynamics of Migration, Health and Livelihoods: INDEPTH Network Perspectives." Aldershotn: Ashgate, 2009.

Consortium for Protecting Refugees and Migrants in South Africa. "Protecting Refugees, Asylum Seekers and Immigrants in South Africa." Johannesburg, South Africa: Consortium for Protecting Refugees and Migrants in South Africa, 2009.

Convention Governing the Specific Aspects of Refugee Problems in Africa. Organization of African Unity Conventions Doc.1001 U.N.T.S. 45, entered into force June 20, 1974.

Cosman, Madeleine. "Illegal Aliens and American Medicine," *Journal of American Physicians and Surgeons*, (2005): 6–10.

Cudd, A., and Robin, A., (Eds.). *Feminist Theory: A Philosophical Approach.* Malden, MA: Blackwell Publishing, 2005.

Dawes, J. "Atrocity and Interrogation." *Critical Inquiry*, 2004: 249–66.

Debusmann, B. "In Mexico's Drug Wars, Bullets and Ballads." *Reuters News Service,* July 9, 2008.

Delaney, P., and Elizabeth, S. "Gender and Post-Disaster Reconstruction: The Case of Hurricane Mitch in Honduras and Nicaragua." *LCSPG/LAC World Bank Gender Team*, January, 2000.

Democracy Now. "Kanye West: 'Bush Doesn't Care about Black People,'" *Democracy Now*, September, 5, 2005. http://www.democracynow.org/2005/9/5/kanye_west_bush_doesnt_care_about (accessed September 20, 2008).

Denzin, N. *Interpretive Ethnography*. Los Angeles, CA: Sage, 2014.

Department of Health and Human Services, United State of America. "Fact Sheet: The Patients' Bill of Rights in Medicare and Medicaid." Accessed April 3, 2013. http://archive.hhs.gov/news/press/1999pres/990412.html

Deutsche Presse-Agentur. "Zimbabwe's Medical Bodies Implore End to Political Violence." *Deutsche Presse-Agentur*, June 6, 2008.

Doucet, A., and Natasha, M. "Feminist Methodologies and Epistemology," in *Handbook of 21st Century Sociology* Edited by Clifton, B., and Peck, D. 36–42. Thousand Oaks, California: Sage, 2006.

Douzinas, C. "Humanity, Military Humanism and the New Moral Order." *Economy and Society*, 2003: 159–83.

Duckett, S. J. *Australian Health Care System*. Melbourne, Australia: Oxford University Press, 2004.

Dugger, C. "In South Africa, an Unlikely Leader on AIDS." *The New York Times,* May 14, 2010.

Economist (*The*) Data Team. "The Toll of a Tragedy." *The Economist* Data Team, July 8, 2015. http://www.economist.com/blogs/graphicdetail/2015/07/ebola-graphics (accesssed July 15, 2015).

Edkins, J. "Sovereign Power, Zones of Indistinction, and the Camp." *Alternatives*, (2000): 3–25.

Emergency Nurses Association. *Triage: Meeting the Challenge*. Park Ridge, IL: Emergency Nurses Association, 1997.

Emergency Nurses Association. *Making the Right Decision: A Triage Curriculum.* Des Plaines, IL: Emergency Nurses Association, 2001.

Enarson, E. "Gender and Natural Disasters." International Labour Office InFocus Programme on Crisis Response and Reconstruction. Geneva: September, 2000.

Enarson, E. "Violence Against Women in Disasters Fact Sheet." School of the Built and Natural Environment, Northumbria University: U.K, 2006.

Enarson, E., Meyreles, L., Gonzalez, M., et al. "Working with Women at Risk: Practical Guidelines for Assessing Local Disaster Risk." International Hurricane Center, Florida International University. Community Risk Assessment and Planning Project, Prevention Consortium, June, 2003.

England, K. V. L. "Getting Personal: Reflexivity, Positionality, and Feminist Research." *The Professional Geographer*, 1994: 80–89.

ESI Triage Research Team & Agency for Healthcare Research and Quality. *Emergency Severity Index Triage Algorithm.* Rockville, MD.: Agency for Healthcare Research and Quality, 2008.

Farris, M. "Study Shows Heavy Health Costs of Katrina." WLTV Eyewitness News, April 3, 2011.

Farmer, P. *Infections and Inequalities: The Modern Plagues.* Los Angeles: University of California Press, 1999.

Farmer, P. "An Anthropology of Structural Violence." *Current Anthropology* (2004): 305–25.

Farmer, P., Bruce N., Stuart S., Keshavjee S. "Structural Violence and Clinical Medicine." *Public Library of Science Medicine*, 3(2006): e449.

Fassin, D. *Humanitarian Reason a Moral History of the Present Times*. Berkeley: University of California Press, 2012.

Fee, E. *Women's Health, Politics, and Power: Essays on Sex/gender, Medicine, and Public Health*. Amityville, N.Y.: Baywood Pub., 1994.

Forced Migration Online. "What is Forced Migration?" Refugee Studies Centre, Oxford University: U.K., 2010. Accessed January 3, 2013. http://www.forcedmigration.org/whatisfm.htm.

Fothergill, A. "Gender, Risk, and Disaster." *International Journal of Mass Emergencies and Disasters*, 1996: 33–56.

Fox News. "Arizona Immigration Enforcement Bill Stirs National Debate." *Fox News*, April 20, 2010.

Freedman, H., and Peter, W. "Protecting Human Rights through International and National Law," in *Social Injustice and Public Health*, Edited by Barry, L., and Victor, S. New York, NY: Oxford University Press, 2006: 480–92.

Freedy, J. R., and Simpson, W. "Disaster-Related Physical and Mental Health: A Role for the Family Physician." *American Family Physician*, 2007: 841–46.

Freemantle, T. "U.S. Immigration: Persecution Claims Open Path for Chinese." *Houston Chronicle*, April 7, 2013.

Fuller, A. "Mandela's Children." *National Geographic*, 217(2010): 80–109.

Furchtgott-Roth, D. "Reduce the High Cost of Medical Malpractice." *Reuters News Services,* 2009.

Galtung, J. "Violence, Peace, and Peace Research." *Journal of Peace Research*, 1969, 167–91.

Galtung, J. "Kulturelle Gewalt." *Der Burger im Staat*. 1993: 106.

Geiger, J. H. "Medical Care," in *Social Injustice and Public Health*, Edited by Barry Levy, S., and Victor, W. S. 207–19. New York, NY: Oxford University Press, 2006.

Giles, W. M., and Jennifer H. (Eds.). *Sites of Violence Gender and Conflict Zones.* Berkeley: University of California Press, 2004.

Gilligan, J. "Violence: Reflections on a National Epidemic." *Vintage,* 1996: 192.

Glaser, D., Christine H., and Michael, J. "Gender Differences in Risk Assessment: Why do Women take Fewer Risks than Men?" *Judgment and Decision Making*, 1(2006): 48–63.

Goldhill, D. "How American Healthcare Killed My Father." *The Atlantic*, September, 2009.

Gunewardena, N., and Mark, S. (Eds.). *Capitalizing on Catastrophe: Neoliberal Strategies in Disaster Reconstruction.* New York, NY: AltaMira Press, 2008.

Hammer, J. "Healing Powers: Africa." *Newsweek*, April 3, 2006. 23–34G.

Hanisch, C. "The Personal is Political," in *Notes from the Second Year: Women's Liberation in 1970*, Edited by Firestone, S. S., and Koedt, A. New York: SCEF, 1969.

Harding, S. "Rethinking Standpoint Epistemology: What is Strong Objectivity?" in *Feminist Epistemologies*, Edited by Alcoff, L. L., and Potter, E. London: Routledge, 1993.

Harding, S. (Ed.). *Feminism and Methodology.* Bloomington: Indiana University Press, 1987.

Harris, G. "Inward, Outward, Onward: Auto-Ethnography of a Dissertation in (Qualitative) Transitional Space." *Qualitative inquiry*, 17(2011): 725–731.

Health and Human Rights Information (HHRI). Gender-Based Violence. 2012. http://www.hhri.org/thematic/gender_based_violence.html (accessed June 4, 2013).

Hodgson, A. "South Africa—The Most Unequal Income Distribution in the World." *Euromonitor International*, June 13, 2012.

House, S., Thérèse, M., and Sue, C. "Menstrual Hygiene Matters: A Resource for Improving Menstrual Hygiene Around the World." London, UK: WaterAid. http://washurl.net/5iyh2e (accessed June 4, 2012).

Harrison, S., Bhana, R., and Ntuli, A., (Eds.). *South African Health Review 2007.* Durban, South Africa: Health Systems Trust, 2007.

Harvey, H. "Rape is Cheaper than Bullets." *The Guardian,* February 24, 2009.

Held, V. *The Ethics of Care: Personal, Political, and Global.* Oxford: Oxford University Press, 2006.

Hesse-Biber, S. N., and Mchelle, Y., (Eds.). *Feminist Perspectives on Social Research.* New York: Oxford University Press, 2004.

Horne, R. "Good Reasons to Believe Worst is Over for Zimbabwe." *Business Day*, July 28, 2009.

Human Rights Watch. "Women's Rights." New York: Human Rights Watch, 2007. http://hrw.org/women (accessed May 12, 2012).

Human Rights Watch. "Neighbors in Need: Zimbabweans Seeking Refuge in South Africa." New York, NY: *Human Rights Watch*, July, 2008.

Institute for Healthcare Improvement. "The Eight Steps to Successful Down Referral: Opening the Door to a PHC- Driven ARV Program." Durban, South Africa: 3rd South African AIDS Conference, June 7, 2007.

Integrated Regional Information Networks. "South Africa's Flawed Asylum System." IRIN: April 30, 2013. Accessed June 14, 2013. http://www.refworld.org/docid/5187a9f74.html

InterAction. *Best Practices for Gender Integration in Organizations and Programs from the InterAction Community*. Washington D.C.: Interaction Publication Commission on the Advancement of Women, U.S. Agency for International Development (USAID), 1998.

International Association for the Study of Forced Migration. *Forced Migration*. Washington D.C.: International Association for the Study of Forced Migration, 2010.

International Convention on the Elimination of all Forms of Racial Discrimination. Adopted by United Nations General Assembly Resolution 2106 (XX) December 21, 1965, Entered into Force January 4, 1969.

International Covenant on Civil and Political Rights. U.N. Document A/6316. Adopted by the U.N. General Assembly Resolution 2200A (XXI) of December 16, 1966, Entered into Force March 23, 1976.

International Covenant on Economic, Social and Cultural Rights. United Nations General Assembly Resolution 2200A (XXI), 21 U.N.GAOR Supp. (No. 16), Entered into Force 3 January 1976.

International Federation of the Red Cross. "The Seven Fundamental Principles." International Federation of the Red Cross, 2010. Accessed February 2, 2012. http://www.ifrc.org/what/values/principles/index.asp.

International Labour Organization. "A Conceptual Framework for Gender Analysis and Planning: Features of the Moser Gender Planning Framework." United Nations, 2013. http: www.ilo.org (accessed May 29, 2014).

International Organization for Migration. "Assessing the Impacts of Migration Policy: An International Comparison." Geneva, Switzerland: International Organization for Migration, 2008.

International Society for Health and Human Rights. "Health and Human Rights Information." 2012. http://www.hhri.org/thematic/gender_based_violence.html (accessed June 12, 2013).

Jackson, J., and John, N. "Health Care Reform Bill Summary: A Look at What's in the Bill." *CBS News*, March 23, 2010.

Jennings, A. "Dying Dad, Jesus Navarro, to get Kidney Transplant Despite Undocumented Immigration Status." *ABC News*, February 8, 2012.

Justice in Mexico Project. "Justice in Mexico Project." University of San Diego, April, 2014.

Kaiser, H. J. Family Foundation. "Health Care Spending in the United States and OECD Countries." Washington, D.C.: Kaiser Foundation, January, 2007.

Kiley, T. Personal Communication, August 31, 2009.

Krieger, N. "Researching Critical Questions in Social Justice and Public Health: An Ecosocial Perspective," in *Social Injustice and Public Health*, Edited by Barry, S. L., and Victor, W. S. 460–79. New York, NY: Oxford University Press, 2006.

Landman, T. *Studying Human Rights*. New York, N.Y.: Routledge, 2006.

Langley, R. *Sex and Gender Differences in Health and Disease*. Durham: Carolina Academic Press, 2003.

LatapÍ, A. E., and Susan, M., (Eds.) *Mexico-U.S. Migration Management: A Bi-National Approach*. Maryland: Lexington Books, 2008.

Levy, B., and Victor, S. *Social Injustice and Public Health*. U.K.: Oxford University Press, 2005.

Lennon, K., and Margaret, W., (Eds.). *Knowing the Difference: Feminist Perspectives in Epistemology*. London, U.K.: Routledge, 1994.

Lewis-Fernández, R., Amar, K. D., César, A., Myrna, M. W., and Mark, O. "Depression in U.S. Hispanics: Diagnostic and Management Considerations in Family Practice." *Journal of the American Board of Family Medicine*, July–August 2005, 282–96.

MacKinnon, C. *Are Women Human?* Harvard University Press, 2006.

Mantilla, K. "Disaster Relief." Female Studies, 2005; 31(3): 679–84.

Mark, S. "Sex- and Gender-Based Medicine: Venus, Mars, and Beyond." Gender Medicine, 2005 September, 2(3): 131–36.

Martin, G. *A Comparative Analysis of the Financing of HIV/AIDS Programmes in Botswana, Lesotho, Mozambique, South Africa, Swaziland and Zimbabwe*. Cape Town, South Africa: The Human Sciences Research Council Press, 2003.

May, C. "Texas Legislator to Mexico: Pay us back!." *The Daily Caller*, April 4, 2012.

Mayo Clinic. "Oral Health: A Window to Your Overall Health." Rochester: Minnesota, 2013. http://www.mayoclinic.com/health/dental/DE00001 (accessed May, 1 2014).

Médecins Sans Frontières. "No Refuge: Medical and Humanitarian Needs of Zimbabweans in South Africa." Johannesburg, South Africa: MSF, June, 2009.

Medicare: U.S. Centers for Medicare & Medicaid Services. "Hospital Compare." Baltimore: Maryland, U.S. Centers for Medicare & Medicaid Services, 2013. http://medicare.gov/hospitalcompare/search.html (accessed February 12, 2014).

Meintjes, S., Anu, P., and Meredeth, T., (Eds.). *The Aftermath: Women in Post-conflict Transformation*. London: Zed Books, 2001.

Meredith, M. *Mugabe: Power, Plunder, and the Struggle for Zimbabwe*. New York, NY: Perseus Books Group, 2007.

Migrant Rights International. "The 1990 Convention." http://www.migrantwatch.org/about_the_convention/Intro.html (accessed May 2, 2014).

Migration Policy Institute. "Mexican Immigration in the U.S." Washington, D.C.: Migration Policy Institute, February, 2010.

Miller-Keane Encyclopedia and Dictionary of Medicine, Nursing, and Allied Health. "Comorbidity." Philadelphia: Saunders, 2003.

Miller, S. "Families of Dead Mexican Illegal Aliens Sue U.S. for $41 Million." *The Washington Times,* May 12, 2012.

Mocellin, J., Thandiwe, M., and Raymond, W. "The Needs of Women in Disasters and Emergencies." Manitoba, Canada: UN Development Programme, June 20, 1994: ix–8.

Mooney, G. "Something is Rotten in SA Hospitals . . . NHI Will Fix It." *Saturday Star*. Johannesburg: April, 7, 2012.

Moser, C. *Gender Planning and Development: Theory, Practice, and Training*. London: Routledge, 1993.

Munakiri, T. "Corruption: Zimbabwe's Biggest Enemy." New Zimbabwe.com. http://www.newzimbabwe.com/pages/opinion225.14972.html (accessed November 12, 2009).

Murry, A. F. *From Outrage to Courage: Women Taking Action for Health and Justice*. Monroe, Me.: Common Courage Press, 2008.

Nagar, R., and Susan, G. "Reflexivity and Positionality in Feminist Fieldwork Revisited," in *Politics and Practice in Economic Geography*, Edited by Adam, T., Eric, S., Jamie, P., and Trevor, B. 267–79. London: SAGE Publications Ltd., 2007.

National Association for the Care of the Handicapped. "Zimbabwe's Medical Bodies Implore an End to Political Violence. Harare: Zimbabwean National Association for the Care of the Handicapped. http://ns1.twocircles.net/2008jun08/zimbabwes_medical_bodies_implore_end_political_violence.html#.U_zdX8J0yM9 (accessed May 26, 2008).

Ndlovu, N. "Immigrants Living with HIV Refused Medication in South Africa." Key Correspondent Team, International HIV/AIDS Alliance: *KC News,* March 6, 2012.

Neacsu, D. "Gender-Based Persecution as a Basis for Asylum: An Annotated Bibliography: 1993–2002." University of Toronto, Law Library, 2013.

Neumayer, E., and Plümper, T. "The Gendered Nature of Natural Disasters: The Impact of Catastrophic Events on the Gender Gap in Life Expectancy 1981–2002." Annals of the Association of American Geographers, 2007(3): 551–66.

Nevarez, G. "Deferred Action Approval Rate Dispute Erupts between Center for Immigration Studies and USCIS." *Huffington Post*, April 29, 2013.

Nussbaum, M. *Women and Human Development: The Capabilities Approach.* New York, NY: Cambridge University Press, 2000.

Nussbaum, M. "Women and Cultural Universals," in *Feminist Theory*, Edited by Cudd, A., and Andreasen, R. 302–24. Malden, MA: Blackwell Publishing, 2006.

O'Connor, M. "How South Africa Became the World's No. 1 Asylum Destination." *The Slate,* August 27, 2010.

Ohlemacher, S. "U.S. Lags Behind 41 Nations in Life Span." *Associated Press*, August 11, 2007.

Office of the Comptroller, Texas. "Undocumented Immigrants in Texas: A Financial Analysis of the Impact to the State Budget and Economy." Austin, TX: Texas Comptroller Carole Keeton Strayhorn. December, 2006.

Pallot, P. "Expat Guide to South Africa: Health Care." *The Telegraph*, May 21, 2010.

Palmary, I., Erica, B., Khatidja, C., and Peace, K. *Gender and Migration Feminist Interventions*. London: Zed, 2010.

Panafrican News Agency. "Cholera: Zimbabwe Report." Panafrican News Agency, February 19, 2010. http://www.afriquejet.com/news/africa-news/cholera-kills-9-in-zimbabwe-2010021744331.html (accessed March 3, 2011).

Pan American Health Organization. "Gender and Natural Disasters." Washington D.C.: Women, Health & Development Program, Pan American Health Organization, 2004.

Patel, V., Melanie, A., Jeremy, B., Charles, T., and Anthony, R. "Depression in Developing Countries: Lessons from Zimbabwe." *Bmj*, 2001, 482–84.

Patients' Bill of Rights Act of 1999. Washington, D.C.: S. 6–106th United States of America Congress, 1999.

Peoplemovin. "Migration Flows Across the World." Peoplemovin.org. http://peoplemov.in/#! (accessed February 27, 2013).

Press Ganey. "Pulse Report 2009: Emergency Department—Patient Perspectives on American Healthcare." Indiana: Press Ganey Associates, Inc., 2009.

Preston, J. "Sharing the Costs Social Composition of Emergency Care." N*ew York Times*, July 18, 2006.

Pulcino, T., Sandro, G., Jennifer, A., Heidi, R., Mary, F., and David, V. "Posttraumatic Stress in Women After the September 11 Terrorist Attacks in New York City." *Journal of Women's Health* 12(2003): 809–20.

Rawls, J. *A Theory of Justice*. Cambridge, M.A.: Harvard University Press, 1971.

Reporters Without Borders. "Mexico." Paris: France, July, 2008. http://www.rsf.org/country-47.php3?id mot=2488&Valider=OK

Reporters Without Borders. "World Report: Mexico." Accessed May 1, 2013. http://en.rsf.org/report-mexico.184.html

Reuters News Service. "Zimbabwe Agrees to IMF Monitoring Programme: Finance Minister." Harare: June 7, 2013.

Richter, R. "Crossing the Gender Divide in Disaster Relief." *Foreign Service Journal* (2006): 41–47.

Richter, R. "Gender Matters: Female-Specific Relief Efforts during Disasters are Key." *Journal of Emergency Medical Services* (2007): 58–63.

Richter, R., and Thomas, F. "Gendered Dimensions of Disaster Care: Critical Distinctions in Female Psychosocial Needs, Triage, Pain Assessment, and Care." *American Journal of Disaster Medicine*, (2008): 31–37.

Roig-Franzia, M. "Discount Dentistry, South of the Border." *Washington Post Foreign Service*, June 18, 2007.

Ruddick, S. "Maternal Thinking," in *Mothering: Essays in Feminist Theory*, ed. Joyce, T. Rowman & Littlefield Publishing, 1980.

Ruiters, G., and Robert van N., (Eds.). *Universal Healthcare in Southern Africa: Policy Contestation in Health System Reform in South Africa and Zimbabwe*. Scottsville, South Africa: University of Kwazulu-Natal Press, 2012.

Sarantakos, S. *Social Research*. Hampshire, U.K.: Palgrave & Macmillan Publishers, 2012.

Sen, A. *Inequality Reexamined.* Cambridge, M.A.: Harvard University Press, 1992.

Seper, J. "Ex-Officer Fights Deportation, Death." *The Washington Times*, March 10, 2009.

Somekh, B., and Cathy, L., (Eds.). *Theory and Methods in Social Research.* Los Angeles, CA: Sage Publications, 2011.

South Africa Constitution. "The Constitution of the Republic of South Africa." Constitutional Court of South Africa: December 4, 1996.

South African Medical Association. "Patient's National Health Rights Charter." South Africa: Department of Health, 2013.

South African Institute of Race Relations. "South Africa Survey 2008/2009," Johannesburg, South Africa: Publication of the SAIRR, 2009.

Stuber, J., Heidi R., and Sandro, G. "Gender Disparities in Posttraumatic Stress Disorder after Mass Trauma." *Gender Medicine*, 3(2006): 54–67.

Sultana, F. "Reflexivity, Positionality and Participatory Ethics: Negotiating Fieldwork Dilemmas in International Research." *ACME: An International E-Journal for Critical Geographies*, 6(2007): 374–85.

Tahirih Justice Center. "Tahirih Wins Key Immigration Case." April 27, 2011. http://www.tahirih.org/2011/04/matter-of-a-t/ (accessed July 1, 2012).

Taylor, A. "Mexico's Drug War: 50,000 Dead in 6 Years." *The Atlantic*, May 17, 2012.

Tena-Tamayo, C. "Malpractice in Mexico: Arbitration Not Litigation." *Bmj*, 2005, 448–51.

The American Heritage Dictionary of the English Language. 3rd ed. Boston: Houghton Mifflin, 1992.

Time Magazine. "Health: The Longest Wait." Time National Survey, November 1, 2004.

Toole, M. "Forced Migrants: Refugees and Internally Displaced Persons," in *Social Injustice and Public Health*, edited by Barry, L., and Victor, S. 190–204. New York, NY: Oxford University Press, 2006.

Transparency International. "Corruption by Country: Mexico." 2012. http://www.transparency.org/country#MEX (accessed August 21, 2103).

Tronto, J. "An Ethic of Care," in *Feminist Theory*, edited by Cudd, A., and Andreasen, R. 251–63. Malden, M.A.: Blackwell Publishing, 2005.

Ullo, J. "Border Violence Brings Asylum Policies into Question." *Brownsville Herald,* April 3, 2010.

UNAIDS/WHO. "2008 Report on the Global AIDS Epidemic." Joint United Nations Programme on HIV/AIDS, July, 2008.

United Nations Development Programme. "Support for Women in Internally Displaced Situations." New York: Report of a Joint Mission of UNDP/UNICEF/WHO/DHA. November, 1993.

United Nations Development Programme. "Gender Development Index." New York: United Nations Development Programme, 2007. Accessed on March 26, 2014. http://hdrstats.undp.org/indicators/269.html

United Nations Development Programme. "Gender Empowerment Measure Report." Human Development Reports. New York, N.Y.: UNDP, 2007. Accessed on March 22, 2013. http://hdrstats.undp.org/indicators/280.html

United Nations General Assembly. "Declaration on the Elimination of Violence against Women." Adopted December 20, 1993, as Res. 48/104.

UNHCR. "Guidelines on the Protection of Refugee Women." Geneva: United Nations High Commission for Refugees, June, 1991.

UNHCR. "What is Mixed Migration?" Regional Mixed Migration Secretariat, Nairobi, Kenya. Accessed on July 26, 2015. http://www.regionalmms.org/index.php?id=60

United Nations Office for the Coordination of Humanitarian Affairs. "Regional Update No. 9 Cholera/Acute Watery Diarrhea Outbreaks in South Africa," Johannesburg: OCHA, April 17, 2009.

United Nations Security Council. Resolution 1325. Adopted by the Security Council at its 4213th meeting, October 31, 2000.

United Nations. United Nations Treaty Collection. New York: 2010. http://treaties.un.org/Pages/ViewDetails.aspx?src=TREATY&mtdsg_no=IV-4&chapter=4&lang=en (accessed May 12, 2012).

United Nations Women. "UN Women Guiding Documents: CEDAW." New York, N.Y., 2013. Accessed on April 1, 2014. http://www.unwomen.org/about-us/guiding-documents

United Nations Women's News. "Challenges by Advocacy Factions." WeNews, March 21, 2013.

United States Department of Health and Human Services—Office of Minority Health. "Hispanic/Latino Health." 2013. Washington, D.C.: Office of Minority Health. Accessed March 12, 2014. http://minorityhealth.hhs.gov/templates/browse.aspx?lvl=2&lvlid=54.

United States Department of Homeland Security & U.S. Citizenship and Immigration Services. "Consideration of Deferred Action for Childhood Arrivals (DACA) Process." 2013. Accessed November 1, 2014. http://www.uscis.gov/portal/site/uscis/menuitem.eb1d4c2a3e5b9ac89243c6a7543f6d1a/?vgnextoid=f2ef2f19470f7310VgnVCM100000082ca60aRCRD&vgnextchannel=f2ef2f19470f7310VgnVCM100000082ca60aRCRD#guidelines.

University of Illinois, Center for Law and Globalization. "Mass Rape." International Criminal Court, 2013.

University of Maine. "The U.S. Healthcare System: Best in the World or Just the Most Expensive?" Bangor, MA: Bureau of Labor Education, 2001.

University of Memphis. "Biopolitics, Biopower, and Life Itself." *Media Theory,* April 14, 2011.

University of Zimbabwe Medical School. "Depression in Developing Countries: Lessons from Zimbabwe." 2001, 482.

Usborne, D. "US Confronts Humanitarian Crisis as Thousands Cross the Texan Border." *The Independent*, June 22, 2014.

USA Today. "Mexico Starts Identifying 72 Massacred Migrants." *USA Today*, August 26, 2010.

Valenzuela, T. D., Spaite, D., Meislin, H., Clark, L. L., Wright, A. L., and Ewy, G. A. "Case and Survival Definitions in Out-of-Hospital Cardiac Arrest." *JAMA*, 1992, 272.

Vearey, J. "Migration, Access to ART, and Survivalist Strategies in Johannesburg." *Journal of AIDS Research* (2008): 361–74.

Wachira, G. "Migrants' Right to Health in South Africa." Johannesburg: Migrant Rights Monitoring Project, Forced Migration Studies Programme, University of the Witwatersrand, 2009.

WaterAid. "Menstrual Hygiene Matters: A Resource for Improving Menstrual Hygiene Around the World." WaterAid and Research Consortium SHARE (Sanitation and Hygiene Applied Research for Equity). November, 2012.

Watson, Cate. "Micropolitics of Desire: Participant Self-Observation, Critical Ethnography and the Return to the Baroque." *Education in the North* (2009): 1–30.

Weist, R., Mocellin, J., and Motsisi, D. "The Needs of Women in Disasters and Emergencies." Winnipeg, Manitoba: Disaster Research Institute, June, 1994.

Wiesenfeld-Hallin, Z. "Sex Differences in Pain Perception." Gender Medicine, 2005 2(3): 137–45.

White House (The). Remarks by the President to a Joint Session of Congress on Health Care. Washington, D.C., U.S. Capitol: Office of the Press Secretary, September, 9, 2009.

Whoriskey, P. "Study Says Storms Displaced More People than Estimated: Poorest Evacuees' Conditions are said to have Worsened." *Washington Post*, August 8, 2007.

Women Human Rights Defenders International Coalition. "Policy Recommendations to Address Critical Security Concerns and Needs of Women Human Rights Defenders in Haiti in the Aftermath of the 12 January Earthquake." Women Human Rights Defenders International Coalition report, February 2, 2010.

World Bank Group. "Moser Gender Analysis Framework and Gender Audit." Poverty and Social Impact Analysis, World Bank, 2012. http://go.worldbank.org/SDR62R2AL0 (accessed March 2, 2013).

World Bank Group. "Vital Gender Statistics not Captured in 90 Percent of Developing World." Washington, D.C.: World Bank, 2007.

World Bank Group. "Women are Less Likely than Men to Participate in the Labor Market in Most Countries." Washington, D.C.: World Bank, Gender and Equality Statistics, September, 4, 2012. http://data.worldbank.org/news/women-less-likely-than-men-to-participate-in-labor-market (accessed October 12, 2012).

World Bank Group. "Ease of Doing Business in Mexico." Washington, D.C.: World Bank, 2013. http://www.doingbusiness.org/data/exploreeconomies/mexico (accessed May 20, 2014).

World Bank Group. "GINI Index." Washington, D.C.: World Bank, 2013. http://data.worldbank.org/indicator/SI.POV.GINI (accessed May 20, 2014).

World Health Organization. "The Right to Health Fact Sheet." Geneva, Switzerland: World Health Organization, August, 2007.

World Health Organization. "World Health Report 2000 Health Systems: Improving Performance." Geneva, Switzerland: World Health Organization, 2000.

World Health Organization. "Gender and Health in Disasters." Geneva, Switzerland: World Health Organization, July, 2002.

World Health Organization. "Effects of Female Genital Mutilation on Childbirth in Africa." Geneva, Switzerland: WHO Department of Reproductive Health and Research, 2008.

World Health Organization. "Wealth, Health and Health Expenditure." NHA Policy Highlight. No. 4, April, 2010.

World Health Organization/UNICEF Joint Monitoring Programme for Water Supply and Sanitation. "Progress on Sanitation and Drinking-Water: 2010 Update." Geneva, Switzerland: World Health Organization, 2010.

World Health Organization. "Drug-Resistant Tuberculosis Now at Record Levels." Geneva, Switzerland: World Health Organization news release, March 18, 2010.

World Health Organization. "Wealth and Health are Correlated." Geneva, Switzerland: World Health Organization, 2003.

World Health Organization. "Spending on Health: A Global Overview." Geneva, Switzerland: World Health Organization, 2004. www.mohcw.gov.zw/index.php/mental-health (accessed May 2, 2013.)

World Health Organization. "UN-Water Global Analysis and Assessment of Sanitation and Drinking Water." Geneva: Switzerland, GLAAS 2012 Report. http://whqlibdoc.who.int/publications/2012/9789241503365_eng.pdf (accessed May 2, 2013).

Worsnip, P. "U.N. Assembly Votes for More Powerful Women's Agency." *Reuters Newswire*, September, 14, 2009.

Yehuda, R. "Immune Neuroanatomic Neuroendocrine Gender Differences in PTSD." Lecture, Program and Abstracts of 154th Annual Meeting of the American Psychological Association, New Orleans, May, 5–10, 2001.

Yonghua, J., Klein, P., Kelton, C., Li, X., and Guo, J. "Utilization and Spending Trends for Antiretroviral Medications in the U.S. Medicaid Program from 1991 to 2005." *AIDS Research and Therapy*, August, 2007.

Zimbabwean Ministry of Health and Child Welfare. "Mental Health," Harare: Zimbabwe, Zimbabwean Ministry of Health and Child Welfare.

Index

Adar, J., 113
Agamben, Giorgio, 21–22, 43

Behar, Joy, 7–8
Bhugra, Dinesh, 117, 128
biopolitics, 16
biosocial research, 16
Bird, Chloe E, 115

CDC-Center for Disease Control, 125, 141
comorbidity/comorbid disease(s), 17
Convention on the Elimination of all Forms of Discrimination Against Women (CEDAW), 38–39
CoRMSA–Consortium for Refugees and Migrants in South Africa, 52, 54, 58, 86, 150
cultural relativism, 44

depression, 131–32
disaster, 17
disaster types, 27

emergency healthcare, 17, 138–39
emergency medicine, 17
EMS–Emergency Medical Services/ Pre-Hospital Care, 17, 87–88
Enarson, Elaine, 29
England, Kim, 5

Farmer, Paul, 2–3, 19, 25, 100
Fassin, Didier, 7, 25
feminist perspectives, 4–7
FGM–Feminine Genital Mutilation, 32–33, 62–63
forced migration/forced migrants, xiv, 18, 29, 163
Furchgott-Roth, Diana, 65

Galtung, Johan, 23–24
GBV–Gender-Based Violence, 17
GDI (Gender-Related Development Index), 34
Geiger, Susan, 5
GEM Gender Empowerment Measure, 34
gender, 17
gender-aware disaster care, 147–50, 159
gender-disaggregated data, 33
Gender Disaster Network/Gender Disaster Resilience Alliance, 144
gender equity/inequity, 3, 154
Giles, W. M., 27, 43
Gilligan, James, 24
GINI Index, 142–43
Goldhill, David, 108
Gunewardena, Nandina, 135–36

Harding, Sandra, 6–7
high versus low acuity, 122–23

HIV/AIDS (AVR and ART), 99, 102, 109, 122
Human Rights Watch, 145
Hyndman, Jennifer, 27, 43

infectious disease, 97

Jones, Peter, 117, 128

Krieger, Nancy, 93–94

Langley, Ricky, 114
Levy, Barry, 114

MacKinnon, Catherine, 44
Médecins Sans Frontières (MSF), 106, 119
Meintjes, Sheila, 30, 138
menstrual hygiene, 126–27
menstruation–medical issues, 127
Meredith, Martin, 8
migration, 18, 48–50
migrants, immigrants, 49
Molyneaux, Maxine, 41
Mooney, Gavin, 86, 142
Moser Gender Planning Framework, 18, 41–42
Mugabe, Robert. 7–8, 49
Munakiri, Tonderai, 9
Myriam Merlet, Anne Marie Coriolan and Magali Marcelin Feminist International Camp, 145

Nagar, Richa, 5
Nussbaum, Martha, 34, 37

Obamacare (Patient Protection and Affordable Care Act of 2010), 7, 108–9

positionality, 18
PTSD–Post-Traumatic Stress Disorder, 31, 117, 128–29
public health/public healthcare, 18, 93

Rawls, J. A., 93
refugee, 18
Reporters without Borders, 10
Richter's "Gender Risk Factors"–Causes & Consequences of Vulnerability, 30–37
Rieker, Patricia Perri, 115
Ruddick, Sara, 43

Sen, Amartya, 37
Shuller, Mark, 135–36
Sidell, Victor, 114
Stevens, M., 113
strategic gender interests (Moser Framework), 18
structuralism, 19
structural violence, 13, 19, 153

Tena-Tamayo, C, 65–66
Transparency International, 10
Triage (ESI and Cape) algorithms, 103
tuberculosis (TB, MDR-TB and XDR-TB), 91, 100

undocumented/unrecognized or illegal refugee/migrant, 19
U.N. High Commissioner for Refugee's Guidelines on the Protection of Refugee Women, 41
Universal Declaration of Human Rights, 11, 38, 55
University of Zimbabwe Medical School, 131
U.N. Women, 39, 143

Vearey, Joann, 117

Wachira, George, 53
WASH (water and sanitation, hygiene), 146
WaterAid, 126
Weist, Raymond, 33
World Bank, 19, 33
World Health Organization's *Gender & Health in Disasters*, 3
World Health Organization's right to health mandate, 92
world health system(s) goals (WHO), 155

About the Author

Roxane Richter, Ph.D., E.M.T. As an E.M.T, Roxane's 15 years of frontline experience in international disaster aid and EMS have provided both the catalyst and the forum for her to research global and gender healthcare disparities. She holds a graduate degree in Cross-Cultural Studies (University of Houston) and a doctorate in Political Studies (University of the Witwatersrand, Johannesburg, South Africa). Roxane is an experienced voice in public health, speaking at World Congress on Emergency Medicine and Disasters, United Nations Association, Amnesty International, and more. Her research has appeared in *International Journal of Mass Emergencies & Disasters, American Journal of Disaster Medicine, Journal of Emergency Medical Services, Foreign Service Journal*, and book chapter "Disparity in Disasters: A Frontline View of Gender-Based Inequities in Emergency Aid and Healthcare" in *Anthropology at the Front Lines of Gender-Based Violence*. Roxane serves as President of World Missions Possible, a nonprofit providing medical care, training, and EMS capacity building to 16 nations. She has traveled to 67 nations, serving with American Red Cross' Disaster Health Services and other nonprofits, providing free medical care to impoverished and disaster-stricken areas.

www.ingramcontent.com/pod-product-compliance
Ingram Content Group UK Ltd.
Pitfield, Milton Keynes, MK11 3LW, UK
UKHW041124071026
15587UKWH00009B/190

9 781498 525442